MIND-BODY CONNECTION
FOR PAIN MANAGEMENT

MIND-BODY
CONNECTION
for Pain Management

Vital Meditation, Mindfulness,
and Movement Techniques to
Ease Chronic Pain

Anna McConville, DPT, PT, PNE

ROCKRIDGE
PRESS

For general information on our other products and services or to obtain technical support, please contact our Customer Care Department within the United States at (866) 744-2665, or outside the United States at (510) 253-0500.

Rockridge Press publishes its books in a variety of electronic and print formats. Some content that appears in print may not be available in electronic books, and vice versa.

Interior and Cover Designer: Mando Daniel
Art Producer: Tom Hood
Editor: Carolyn Abate
Production Editor: Matthew Burnett

Illustrations courtesy of Shutterstock (cover, interior).
Author photograph courtesy of Autumn Lee

ISBN: Print 978-1-64739-951-1 | eBook 978-1-64739-562-9

R0

For Steve, who patiently learned the science and healing techniques as I wrote this book; and for my father, who taught me to keep looking for solutions.

Contents

Introduction

The doctor patted me on the shoulder as he led me to the door. "Don't worry, honey," he said. "You're young, and back pain is the most common thing in the world. You'll just have to learn how to live with it."

I had just flown in from California, taking a break from the international mime and comedy school where I spent my days learning how to juggle, do trapeze work, and circus performing. Only at that moment, I couldn't walk a block without crying from the pain. I went to bed that night praying to die. (Yes, the drama of youth.) But I did wake up—in pain and mad as hell that someone was telling me that I wasn't going to be able to live my life the way I wanted.

Determined to not accept the inevitable that I was told, I went to the local library to do some research. I checked out every book I could find on pain, meditation, diet, and exercise. As I began to devour their information, I started to understand how my emotions and stress were tied to my pain. I also learned that I could begin to improve if I moved just a little bit every day and then a little bit more the next.

That's when I began the practice of daily meditation. Confession: I have the most active, busy, convoluted mind of anyone I know. So the fact that I could learn how to quiet my mind and find some sort of peace made me realize that this was possible for others. Because of what I gleaned, I was able to return to my career and travel around the country with a three-person pantomime and clown troupe. That is, until one summer, when I decided to enroll.

That began my 40-year journey of research and practice in holistic health care. I am a complete devotee of mind over matter. Back in 1978, when I was accepted into a very competitive physical therapy program, integrating body and mind practices in therapies wasn't the standard—but I did it anyway. Even now, I'm still a bit of an outlier in the medical field—but things are changing rapidly. I specialize in complex conditions, working with people who haven't had success in traditional methods of care. I've always tried to think of myself as a steward of hope as I walk with my patients through their pain journey, in search of relief.

I believe that we're often given situations that make us stronger. My own continued pain saga drives me to maintain the mindset that I have control over my pain, and that I have tools to help me stay in control. I'm excited to share some of these techniques with you.

The exercises and tips in this book are derived from my own work and that of the many mentors in my journey to wellness. For each and every one of them, I've drawn on the ancient wisdom of healing through the mind-body connection. My favorite third-grade teacher, Sister Genevieve, told me that there was nothing new under the sun. That comment resonated with me as I was writing this book. You may notice that some of the exercises seem familiar, but they are now presented with pain relief in mind. While they may not be new, you are free to change up the exercises to make them fun and make them yours.

The exercise chapters are divided into five different types of mind-body exercises: reframing, mindfulness, meditation, breathwork, and restorative yoga. You'll learn about each one and then you'll be asked to do some exercises. Don't worry if you don't like all of the exercises, because there are plenty to try. And who knows, maybe you'll end up revising some to fit your sensibilities.

This book is here to help you find the right exercises and gain control of your pain by integrating your mind and body. Each chapter has a variety of exercises that range from simple to slightly complex. Each exercise uses mind-body connections to help you feel, breathe, and move in new ways that will change up your routines. The more you understand how pain and stress impact your body, the easier it is for you to be creative and expand on the exercises.

There are no rules about how to read the book or follow the exercises. The most important thing is to be consistent—give them a try and see how they feel. This book isn't meant to be a replacement for seeing a physician or any other health care provider. It's intended to empower you to know that we all have to advocate for our own health.

Remember, self-care *is* health care.

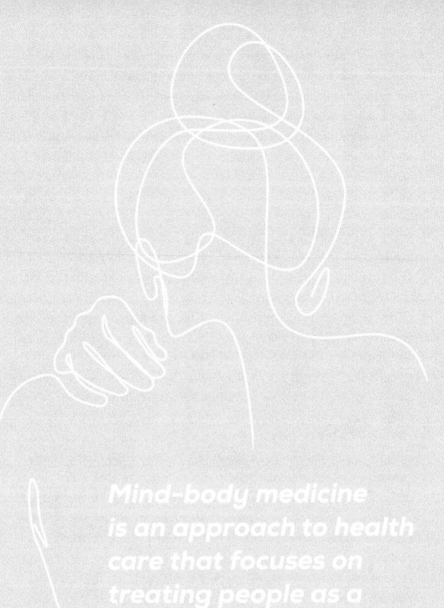

Mind-body medicine is an approach to health care that focuses on treating people as a totality of mind, body, consciousness, spirit, and soul.

CHAPTER ONE

Using the Mind-Body Connection to Manage Pain

In this chapter, you're going to learn about the mind-body connection (MBC) and how it can benefit you. You'll also discover the science behind it and how to identify different types of pain. Then I'll walk you through the various techniques you'll be using in this book to integrate the MBC into your life.

What the Mind-Body Connection Can Do for You

There are a lot of options today for people who want to ease or control the physical pain they experience. Perhaps you've tried physical or chiropractic therapy, or taken various medications. Maybe you've even had surgery. Even after all of these tried-and-true medical solutions, you might still find yourself dealing with a stiff back, a sore ankle, inflammation in your wrists. Perhaps you have migraine headaches that go on for days. Whatever is ailing you, I want you to know that you are not alone.

According to the Centers for Disease Control and Prevention (CDC), in 2016, nearly 25 percent of people in the United States have experienced chronic pain. That's about one in 10 people. This translates to a cost of more than $560 billion in medical care, lost wages, and disability programs.

Whatever brought you here, to the pages in this book, the fact that you are reading it shows that you're ready to try new approaches to better manage your pain. I know from my personal experience—as well as decades of helping patients with complex, multifaceted pain—that the exercises in the coming pages are powerful ways to manage pain.

Mind-body medicine is an approach to health care that focuses on treating people as a totality of mind, body, consciousness, spirit, and soul. This type of treatment is an awareness that our emotions, thoughts, behavior, social surroundings, and spiritual beliefs all affect our health and well-being.

It's clear that the brain and the neurological, endocrine, and immune systems all communicate with one another; there is no real division between the mind and the body. Practicing medicine through the mind-body lens is now more mainstream than ever before, because science now knows that our thoughts and feelings create a chemical response in the body, which can then create physical and physiological changes.

When you are exercising, for example, your brain produces its own chemicals called endorphins and enkephalins as a part of a complex system for regulating pain and managing mood. You've probably heard of the runner's high—that feeling of euphoria, energy, and reduced pain that many people experience after they've engaged in a long stint of aerobic activity. I find it amazing that with only a little bit of effort, we can begin making our own "drugs" to manage pain! My favorite saying that is used extensively in the pain and neuroscience world is "motion is lotion." Our bodies and brains have a beautiful relationship with each other. What we think affects who we are in one big, beautiful, human package.

THE MIND-BODY CONNECTION THROUGH THE AGES

The concept of the mind-body connection has been around for many generations. About 300 years ago, most medical systems throughout the world treated the mind and body as a whole. But during the seventeenth century, the Western world started to see the mind and body as two distinct entities. In the 1600s, Sir Isaac Newton popularized the idea of curing illness with science. The discoveries of bacteria and, later, antibiotics led many doctors to believe that the mind had nothing to do with curing an ailment or illness. Basically, this new science created a separation of human spiritual and emotional dimensions from the physical body. Matters of the mind, soul, and spirit were left to the church, while doctors and scientists took care of the body.

In the past century, however, this compartmentalization has started to change. Researchers began to study

CONTINUED

the MBC and demonstrate the scientific links between the body and mind. While working as an army medic in World War II, anesthesiologist and ethicist Henry Beecher witnessed the power of placebo. When the supply of life-sustaining morphine ran out, he replaced it with a simple saline solution. But since the soldiers thought that it was morphine, their bodies responded as though they were being treated with the powerful drug. In the late twentieth century, neuroscientist Candace Pert, Ph.D., led discoveries showing that the brain makes its own morphine-like substances in the form of endorphins, which exist throughout the entire body.

Even so, the greater medical community—and society in general—has taken its time embracing MBC as true, preventive medicine. According to a study published in the peer-reviewed journal EMBO Reports, in the 1980s, when doctors began emphasizing lifestyle changes—meditation, yoga, stress management, and a low-fat diet—to prevent heart disease, that approach wasn't taken seriously until further studies could confirm the efficacy of the theory. Luckily, these MBC techniques were shown to improve health, and are now considered the hallmark for preventive medicine to maintain good heart health.

Fast-forward to current times, and we now see the country's leading medical institutions and medical schools all incorporating some type of MBC solutions in their treatment plans, including Yale, the University of California System, Mayo Clinic, and Johns Hopkins. In fact, you may have already heard of some of the terms used in MBC techniques: yoga, Pilates, meditation, and even simple long walks. In fact, you may already practice these MBC techniques—you just didn't know it!

Benefits of the Mind-Body Connection

One of the biggest benefits of the MBC is that it's free and at our fingertips anytime and anyplace. It's a vital—and affordable—tool for pain management. Awareness of your MBC can help you cope better with illness and chronic pain, and speed up your recovery. Research tells us that our emotions impact the chemicals in our body, which impact our ability to manage pain and stress. What we do with our physical body—such as posture and exercise—influences how we perceive our well-being and livelihood.

Take a minute to notice your posture right now. Are you sitting up straight? If so, slouch down. Notice how that feels. Now, sit tall and take a deep breath. Feel any different? You have an intricate connection between your body and your mind that can easily be shifted with your awareness and attention.

Good health impacts your brain, which impacts your sleep. A lack of sleep can negatively affect your gut, which in turn affects the production of the chemicals that course through your body. This change in your hormones can influence how you manage pain and stress. Being mindful of how the MBC influences the different aspects of your life helps you move closer to managing your pain in the most impactful ways.

Take Charge of Your Healing

Knowledge is power. The techniques that you'll learn to use for pain management give you control over how you heal and how you feel.

Research shows that mind-body medicine can help rewire your nervous system, helping you steer yourself away from pain and into comfort. Of course, that rewiring takes time, but that time is your own. You don't need to go to an appointment to practice MBC techniques. Even better, you can do the exercises in the comfort of your own home, and even in your pajamas if you like. Even so, before you get started please talk to your doctor or therapist about any plans to integrate MBC techniques into your care program.

There's no right or wrong way to do any of the exercises that you'll be learning. The beauty of using these techniques is that you can be as creative as you want. If you're a morning lark, you can do these exercises as soon as you get up. If you're more of a night owl, you can practice MBC techniques in the evening or right before bed. I'll talk about self-motivation in a later chapter, but the important thing is to feel comfortable doing the exercises and to use them enough long enough to see if they will work for you. No two people are alike, so you have the unique opportunity to create your own sustainable and effective exercises for pain relief.

As you begin to try out these practices, you'll discover that some techniques may work better for you or simply resonate more than others. In other words, you may have a friend who swears by yoga's healing powers, but perhaps you'll discover that breathwork is what seems to work best for you.

Because there are so many MBC techniques to help you manage your pain, I encourage you to give them all a try. If you can, take some notes so that you can remember how you feel after the different practices. You'll start to notice which ones work best for you. At the same time, if you find yourself getting in a rut with some of the exercises you can switch it up. The variety of exercises I've collected here really puts you in charge of finding the right method to help ease discomfort and reduce your pain.

Use the Body to Your Advantage

Medication, surgery, and therapy for pain management all come at a price, whether it's psychological, physical, or financial. That's not to say that medication or health care within the system isn't important. If you break a leg, you need a cast to help you heal. Medications that calm nerves or help with depression are all important tools that help you feel better. But you also have the power to learn new techniques and develop an awareness within. MBC doesn't look outward for solutions—it's an inward journey that allows you to tap into your own internal wisdom for self-care.

Learning to harness that energy in a way that helps you ease whatever physical discomfort or pain you experience will give you a sense of agency that you can't get from external sources. Using your mind—how you think, what you focus on—to help manage your pain can be a profound endeavor—one that can bring about positive, life-long implications. What's more, once you've figured out techniques that work well to ease your pain, you'll also begin to feel the positive effects on your emotional well-being and outlook. It's a true win-win arrangement for both your physical and emotional health—one that you will play a part in achieving.

Preventive Measures and Fewer Side Effects

In essence, the MBC exercises in this book are designed to help in two key areas in your life: The first is to maintain wellness while preventing illness and injury, and the other is to help you find relief in a more holistic and integrative manner. Regular use of these exercises may help you stave off serious complications as a result of acute or chronic pain. They can also be integrated in your recovery plan as you work with your doctor and healthcare practitioners. You may find it useful to use some of these techniques to prepare for or even avoid surgery.

For argument's sake, let's say that you do elect to have surgery to help with a chronic pain issue. What follows is weeks of recovery. Most likely you'll be holed up in your home or in a rehabilitation center to restore your balance and stability with the help of medical professionals. Once you get the green light to move around, you'll need equipment to help you walk and maybe a handicap placard for easier parking. And did I mention weeks and weeks of physical therapy, plus more time off work for recovery at home? There is no question that the cost of surgery, medications, and time off work has an enormous financial impact.

Let's be clear: This book shouldn't take the place of professional medical advice. But I am encouraged to see more medical professionals embrace more holistic approaches to managing pain before diving into medication or surgery to help ease patients' chronic discomfort. Using MBC as part of your self-healing program—after surgery or in conjunction with other recovery protocols—is a prudent path. It can help bring about keen awareness as you begin your journey toward healing.

Using MBC techniques as a means to prevent serious injury is an equally important method. Maybe you experience a sore back after a difficult night's sleep or a stiff hip after a long walk. Perhaps you suffer from slight inflammation in your wrists after a long day in front of a computer. When you start to notice these types of aches and pains with consistency, your body is telling you it isn't happy about your conditions. Learning to use MBC tools takes time and repetition, but when followed correctly, they can help alleviate long-term side effects after major surgery, or prevent small aches and pains from expanding and eventually leading to surgery.

The Science Behind the Mind-Body Connection

Your mind is more powerful than you might realize. How you feel and what you think directly affect your body by changing the structure of your brain and how your immune system functions. Feelings such as gratitude, happiness, and joy have been shown to change the brain in areas that control higher-level thinking. The same can be said for feelings of anger, frustration, and stress. These negative feelings can also alter the pathways in your brain and ultimately influence what occurs in your body.

A 2016 study on meditation published in *Biological Psychiatry* showed that the practice can change the structure of the brain and the workings of the immune system. The study participants were considered "stressed job-seeking unemployed adults." They participated in either a three-day intensive residential mindfulness meditation program or a relaxation training program. After the study, blood tests from the participants revealed reduced levels of inflammation in those who meditated compared with those who didn't.

Inflammation contributes to chronic conditions such as Alzheimer's, arthritis, heart disease, and diabetes. Further research indicates that positive emotions can help reduce harmful levels of stress hormones and even affect your gene susceptibility to different diseases. That's why it's just as important to work on your brain as your body.

The more you feel positive emotions—or even neutral emotions, such as when you meditate—the better you can learn how to control the negative emotions, such as fear and worry. Learning to mitigate your negative emotions when you experience a stressful or frustrating situation can help you become more resistant to infection, inflammation, and disease.

Hardwired Reactions and Connections

You can sit in a chair, not moving a muscle, and simply think a thought that has to do with feeling angry, sad, or happy. Suddenly your pancreas secretes a hormone that affects your blood sugar. Next your liver makes an enzyme, your spleen is sending a message to your thymus gland, your blood is flowing in your capillaries, and your skin changes. All of this happened with a single thought. Your nervous system does this automatically when you're in danger, because you are always instinctively scanning your environment in order to survive.

The autonomic nervous system is made up of both the sympathetic system—which triggers the fight-or-flight response—and the parasympathetic system, which manages rest and repair. The brain sends a message down your body into organs, muscles, glands, and blood. The sympathetic nervous system kicks into action when you have—or think you have—an emergency. This is your vigilance scanning system. When somebody startles you, your sympathetic nervous system releases adrenaline, which causes your stomach to clench, your heart to race, and your sweat glands to activate. You are suddenly shaky and emotional. All this happens as result of chemical messengers that are affecting your body. Your brain made these hormones automatically on the fly. An amazing superpower of the brain is that if you were to think about this startling event in detail again later, the brain would produce those same stress chemicals.

Pain is predominantly influenced by what we think, and is generated entirely in the brain. Like an alarm, it lets us know that there is danger, but there's no information about the extent of that danger. So we use our thoughts, history of pain, and emotions to help us determine how dangerous this pain threat might be, regardless of whether it actually exists.

Positive Influences of MBC

Now that you understand how stress in the fight-or-flight response can create distress in the body, let's look at how using MBC can tap into a chain reaction that produces positive outcomes.

Weight loss. Losing weight via exercise reduces pressure on your knee joints and can relieve compression that exacerbates pain from rheumatism and arthritis. Exercise produces serotonin and dopamine, which help the natural pharmacy in the brain to release its equivalent to morphine.

Stress and anxiety. Anxiety produces hormones such as cortisol, which is a factor in weight gain and abdominal fat. When increased abdominal fat is present, the risk for heart attacks, strokes, and other chronic health conditions is higher. Stress is one of the leading causes of all medical visits, and chronic stress is linked to microscopic changes in the brain that are associated with depression and mental illness. Stress can also suppress the immune system, increasing susceptibility to illness. By positively managing stress through the MBC, we can help boost our immune systems.

Sleep. Insomnia is an epidemic, and sleep can be a complex subject. Poor sleep impacts the brain, the body, and mental health. Using MBC tools, you can improve your ability to sleep, which impacts all aspects of your life. In an interview for *The Guardian*, neuroscientist Matthew Walker, Ph.D., said, "No aspect of our biology is left unscathed by sleep deprivation. It sinks down into every possible nook and cranny. And yet no one is doing anything about it." A consistent good night's sleep improves learning and also protects your heart, brain, well-being, and ability to maintain proper weight. Sleep hygiene is a learned behavior, and it involves many of the tools found in this book.

Identifying Pain

Pain and stress go hand in hand. Everyone experiences stress—it's a natural part of life. But too much stress can lead to many negative effects on the body and mind. In addition to the psychological impact of stress, research has shown that it can exacerbate many chronic conditions, such as acid reflux, asthma, eczema, chronic pain, and headaches.

Symptoms and side effects of stress are one of the most prevalent reasons that people seek health care. According to the National Institutes of Health (NIH), an estimated 31 percent of all adults experience anxiety disorder at some time in their life, while the CDC reported that, in 2018, 50 million Americans had severe chronic pain. That's more than 20 percent of the adult population who are limited in their lives and work.

Acute Pain Versus Chronic Pain

MBC techniques address the biopsychosocial components of both acute and chronic pain, which are very different.

Acute pain is usually sharp, sudden, and specific. While horrible to experience, it lets us know that we need to rest our body. Acute pain often accompanies surgery, dental work, childbirth, or a sprained ankle. This is when medication, crutches, and rest are important. After six months, you should expect tissues to fully heal. Acute pain doesn't generally last longer than six months, and goes away when there is no longer an underlying cause.

Chronic pain is ongoing and can continue even though the tissue has healed. Ongoing pain is a result of a sensitive nervous system. It's multifactorial, meaning that there's more than tissue damage occurring—the whole body and brain become more sensitive. Examples of chronic pain include headaches, osteoarthritis, back pain, fibromyalgia, and collagen diseases. Chronic pain can cause a whole cascade of biopsychosocial events, impacting the body, mind, and spirit.

Chronic pain can become coupled with fear of movement, fear of job loss, and a chain of emotional thoughts about what might happen if you continue to hurt. Physical effects include tense muscles, as well as stress and anxiety about the impact of ongoing pain. In this instance, "motion is lotion."

But the difficult part of moving with pain is convincing your frightened brain that doing so will improve your situation. After all, pain is real! Your brain has determined that there is pain, and your body responds to that information. Fortunately, MBC techniques can help your system become less sensitive to the alarms that are causing your chronic pain.

Nerve Pain

The body has billions of nerve cells that are connected like highways. The nervous system is a living, breathing alarm system that sends danger messages in order to keep you safe. Take, for example, when you step on a sharp rock. The nerve in that leg sends a message to your brain that there is danger under your foot, and you better pay attention The brain gets your attention, and you hop off the offending rock, sit down, and rub your foot. Once you've done that, the alarm in your brain should relax and go back to normal. But for some people, this alarm is extra sensitive. This continued pain can even cause the neighboring nerves to become more sensitive.

When you experience nerve pain, or neuropathic pain, the messages coming to your brain are extra sensitive. Imagine a house alarm system that goes off when a leaf blows against the door. Remember, pain is real, and the information that's coming into your brain is letting you know that you have some sort of crisis to respond to in your nervous system. Medication can calm the nerve cell, or calm your brain to let it know to not be so worried about the incoming information. When you can calm the nervous system, you reset your alarm and decrease the pain message.

Nerve pain can be due to problems in the central nervous system, which includes the brain and spinal cord, or in the nerves that connect to the muscles and organs. Although nerve pain is generally caused by injury or disease, in some cases nerve pain develops for no apparent reason.

Certain words that I hear from my patients help me understand that they are talking about nerve pain; examples include *shooting, stabbing, burning, tingling, throbbing,* and *electrical shocks.* They may be dropping things or falling because their sensation isn't intact. This tells me that they are dealing with a nerve problem. If you suffer from chronic pain, you may have some of these common nerve pain sensations. These are only a few examples of the many ways that nerve pain can impact your health:

Diabetes. About 30 percent of neuropathic pain comes from diabetes. This can manifest as intense burning and aching pain in your feet.

Migraines. These intense headaches can cause sharp, throbbing, or pulsing pain.

Carpal tunnel syndrome. This debilitating nerve condition causes tingling, numbness, and pins-and-needles pain.

Cancer or viral infections such as the flu. These can cause deep aching, stabbing, burning, numbness, and hot or cold sensitivity.

Autoimmune disorders. Lupus, Lyme disease, rheumatoid arthritis, fibromyalgia, shingles, and spinal stenosis can cause intense burning, stabbing, and aching pain, as well as temperature sensitivity.

Tissue Pain

Nociceptive pain is caused by injury to the tissue, including on and under the skin and in the organs. Sensors called nociceptors provide a lot of information. They respond to physical, temperature, and chemical stressors. An example of a physical stressor would be sitting on a hard chair for hours, which sends information from your glutes to your spinal cord to your brain that you'd better get up and move to get some blood flowing. A temperature sensor would tell you to pull your hand away from a flame, because you've learned it may burn you. Chemical sensors are the chemicals your body produces due to inflammation, stress, and even happiness.

Nociception is a good thing because it makes us aware of what's happening to our tissues, joints, and organs. Types of tissue pain include:

Bone fractures. Sensors in bones are highly aware of stresses and strains. If you've ever broken a bone, you know how much pain it can cause. But if you've got a cast on that broken bone, often that pain goes away, or is not as severe when the limb is supported.

Bursitis. This is a type of inflammatory tissue pain. In the inflammatory fluid, you'll find chemicals that irritate your nerve endings. It's kind of like hot pepper in soup—spicy and disruptive to the system.

Muscle strain. When you strain a muscle, it sends a message to the brain that there is pain, and it causes swelling. Other muscles around the strained one get tighter to support the injury so that the body can heal itself.

Inflammation. Autoimmune diseases such as rheumatoid arthritis and gout are characterized by pain, swelling, tenderness, and warmth in the joints. The fluid that surrounds the joint contains a chemical that causes irritation to the nerve and surrounding tissues.

Organ pain. People often wonder if they can feel organ pain. Of course—organs have sensors on them as well. When you have a bladder infection, for instance, you may find that your lower back is achy. Cancer can also cause organ pain depending on which organ it's residing in.

In my practice, I talk about red flags. When somebody describes the pain in the right shoulder and my exam shows me that their shoulder is perfectly fine, I may wonder about lung cancer. Or pelvic pain may be an indicator of prostate cancer. This is the beauty of the nociception alarm system in the body: It keeps us alert in our day-to-day activities that something might be going on to which we should pay attention.

Depression, Anxiety, and Pain

Remember, pain is ultimately a chemical reaction that takes place when your brain deciphers information coming in from your body. When pain is prolonged, it affects the chemical balance that helps your body stay calm, and prevents oversensitivity of the nervous system. When pain overstays its welcome, depression and anxiety are sometimes—and often likely—not far behind.

When we are healthy, our brains are able to produce pain relievers that are more powerful than anything we can buy. But when ongoing pain causes the body to use up all of these pain-relieving chemicals, it depletes the body's ability to create the chemical soup necessary for soothing properties. Essentially there aren't enough of the right chemicals to soothe the body.

Depression and anxiety can be the result of that chemical depletion because the body is now low on "feel-good" pain relievers. Thoughts and worries—these are nerve impulses. So, the more you worry, the more active your detrimental brain chemicals are on the body.

When you are healthy, your brain is able to produce powerful pain relievers. Your family history and your environment also play a role in how well you make these chemicals. These conditions are ultimately considered "chemical" even though they are in essence, "feelings," because they influence the chemical imbalance coursing through your body that affects your pain.

Pain that's impacted by increased mental, emotional, and behavioral factors is called psychogenic pain. It's important to understand that even though this type of pain may arise from a nonphysical source, it's a very real pain and needs to be taken seriously. Examples of this are stomach pain, headache, and back pain. Perhaps you've noticed that when you have more stress, anxiety, or depression, you're more prone to experiencing increased back pain and even headaches.

It's easy to understand how back pain can cause depression and anxiety; it is often so debilitating that it can prevent you from engaging in social and physical activity. But the relationship between stomach pain and your mental health is much more complex.

The digestive system, or gut system, is home to the microbiome. Here your body produces up to 70 percent of your serotonin—the feel-good chemical—and it's also where 80 percent of your immune system resides. If your gut is out of balance, it can affect the chemicals in your brain and put your entire body out of balance, leading to depression and anxiety. As you can see, the correlation between pain and anxiety and depression is cyclical; pain can cause depression, and depression can cause pain.

This is why MBC tools are an excellent source of relief for pain—no matter the cause or origin. They tap both the mind and physical body to release those feel-good chemicals, so you can soothe and heal from within.

CHRONIC PAIN BY
THE NUMBERS

More than 100 million Americans have some sort of persistent or chronic pain. The NIH estimates that at least 20 million people have what is called high-impact pain, which is severe enough to affect everyday lives. Lower back pain is one of the most common types of chronic pain. Women, the elderly, and poor and rural populations are at the highest risk of developing persistent pain, according to the CDC. Add to those facts an aging population in the United States and the problem is only getting worse.

All these issues culminate in health care expenditures that, in the United States, far exceed those in other countries. Turns out treating pain is profitable. New research, published in the *Journal of the American Medical Association* in 2018, shows that the United States spends twice as much on health care as any other high-income country in the world. Using fancy imaging technology such as MRI and CT scans was a contributing factor.

But the growing prevalence of persistent pain research has shown that teaching patients about pain helps decrease the cost of treating it by putting the control back in the patients' hands. A 2016 article in the *Journal of Spine Surgery* revealed that pain education led to a 45 percent savings in health care costs over one year and a 37 percent savings over three years. All this indicates that investing in self-care and education can be just as beneficial. Even large institutions like Veterans Affairs have begun exploring the benefits and cost savings of incorporating MBC into the health care system.

Mind-Body Techniques

MBC is an individualized practice. You may have identified with some of the previously mentioned examples, and by now you should realize that pain is about utilizing the mind to soothe and find relief. What we think affects how we feel. How we feel affects how we think.

The MBC techniques that you're going to learn in this book are coping strategies and stress-management techniques that will allow you to manage your pain, and become a partner in your own healing. For the purposes of this book, you will focus on five different practices that will allow you to find a new way to think, move, and feel.

Reframing Your Thoughts

Reframing thoughts involves changing your perspective on the situation to make it more meaningful, neutral, or positive to you. When you reframe your thoughts about pain, you create a powerful coping technique. With pain, there's often an element of fear about how long it will last and how disabling it may be. Reframing—sometimes called cognitive restructuring—is part of cognitive behavioral therapy. It's a coping technique that you can do at home or with help from a remote therapist. It teaches you to take control of your thoughts and understand that what you think is not necessarily true.

Reframing takes practice—it's like developing a mental muscle that you need to teach yourself to use over and over to strengthen it. But with consistent use, it becomes much easier. And before you know it you'll develop the ability to catch yourself in the act of creating a thought that isn't helpful. As Viktor Frankl said: "Everything can be taken from a man but one thing: the last of the human freedoms—to choose one's attitude in any given set of circumstances." This approach is a key aspect to the MBC.

Mindfulness

The root concept for the word *mindfulness* stems from the word *sati*, in the ancient Indian language of Pali. Loosely translated, the word means "awareness." That means noticing things for what they are without adding or subtracting anything. You observe your thoughts, sensations in the body, and emotions in a neutral way—all without judgment. Mindfulness is a process of living in the present moment. Another way to think of it is as if you are getting into the zone or hitting the pause button.

The roots of mindfulness date back to the beginnings of Buddhism. It became more popular in the United States in the 1960s when Thích Nhất Hạnh, a Buddhist Zen master and poet, introduced his teachings. He wrote that the fatigue that grips many of us at the end of the workday is not natural tiredness. Instead, it's the product of a day filled with wasted thought and feelings of anxiety and worry, as well as anger and resentment. He believed that these negative mental states did more to sap energy than anything else. In the late 1970s, Jon Kabat-Zinn founded mindfulness-based stress reduction. Originally it was designed for the chronically ill, but it quickly became popular in business, health care, and schools.

Mindfulness views negative emotions as part of the normal human experience. It allows you to experience your thoughts, rather than actively—and quickly—reframing them, as we do when sad or hurtful feelings come up. Both mindfulness and reframing are part of attitude/thought-awareness techniques geared toward decreasing your stress and maintaining a calm mind and body. Quite simply, mindfulness is the act of bringing your full consciousness to the present moment, and observing with all of your senses what's around you and what's inside you. Learning to observe in an objective way takes time and practice, but it's free and available anytime and anyplace.

Meditation

Meditation is often used in the same breath as mindfulness, but there are differences. Mindfulness is the act of being present in the moment, and can be practiced anywhere. If you had a pain in your knee, for example, you would notice that pain and not judge that pain. Meditation, on the other hand, is a more formalized practice done at a specific time in a specific place. It's usually practiced in a comfortable position, with an awareness of your breath, and by guiding your mind to stillness.

Harvard psychologists Matthew A. Killingsworth and Daniel T. Gilbert found that people spend nearly 47 percent of their waking hours thinking about something other than what they are doing. Day dreaming isn't inherently bad, but preoccupation can get in the way of productivity or progress. Just 10 minutes of meditation a day for two weeks has been proven to increase the areas of the brain that help with emotional regulation and focus. The parts of the brain used in meditation practice increase in size and undergo neural rewiring, or so-called regrowth, more commonly known as neural plasticity.

There are a many of types of meditation practices, including visualization, guided, loving-kindness, breath awareness, Zen, and vipassana meditation. Dr. Herbert Benson, well known for his relaxation response research and its effect on our physiology, said that "all you need is a quiet space, a comfortable position, a receptive attitude, and the mental device or 'meditation broom' to sweep clean the corners of your mind." When used in conjunction with mindfulness, meditation is an essential tool to help reduce pain through MBC.

Breathwork

Breathwork is a term for a variety of breathing practices in which you consciously control your breathing to affect your mental, emotional, or physical state. It has evolved to include many techniques that focus breathing exercises as a means of self-healing.

The connection between breath, mind, and spirit—and using breath to attain different states of consciousness—dates back to preindustrial civilizations, and you'll find breathwork in many different traditional cultures. The similarity is that these cultures consider the concept of breath as both the act of taking physical air into the lungs, and the spiritual life force that creates life.

There are many styles of breathwork. Pranayama is controlling your breath to move past emotional and energy blocks that inhibit your life flow. Holotropic breathwork involves inhaling and exhaling for the same amount of time and at different speeds to induce an altered state of consciousness. Rebirthing breathwork incorporates circular breathing, sometimes underwater, that creates a state of relaxation that releases pent-up stress.

The most common breathing technique, diaphragmatic breathing, is our most natural way of breathing. Watch your pets or babies—this is how they breath. Unfortunately, Americans have been taught to pull in our bellies and tighten our belts. During sleep we revert back to our natural abdominal breathing patterns. Breathwork is used in both mindfulness and meditation practices. Conscious breathing techniques affect both the brain and the body. Circular breathing can increase serotonin and dopamine release, as well as enhance alpha brain activity, which creates a relaxed, calm sensation. This change in brain chemistry helps increase relaxation, mental clarity, and emotional regulation.

Restorative Yoga

The word *yoga* comes from Sanskrit, meaning "to yoke," as in "to harness." Restorative yoga, based on the work of B. K. S. Iyengar, incorporates props, tools, and modified poses to help prevent pain in people who are recovering from illness or injury. It is often thought of as active relaxation and is also called the rest-and-digest practice. In restorative yoga, the body is supported with props such as towels, bolsters, and pillows, using gravity to assist in relaxation and release of tension. It's usually done in a dark room with silence, warmth, and breathing techniques to calm the mind.

The props allow you to hold poses for longer periods of time while giving your muscles time to relax deeply. This is unlike the majority of yoga classes, which are an active practice. Restorative classes are slow and gentle, making them ideal for people who are experiencing pain and stress. Research into restorative yoga has found that it can alleviate symptoms of anxiety, depression, and pain. Common benefits include relieving the effects of chronic stress, decreased blood pressure, improved sleep and digestion, and decreased muscle tension and fatigue.

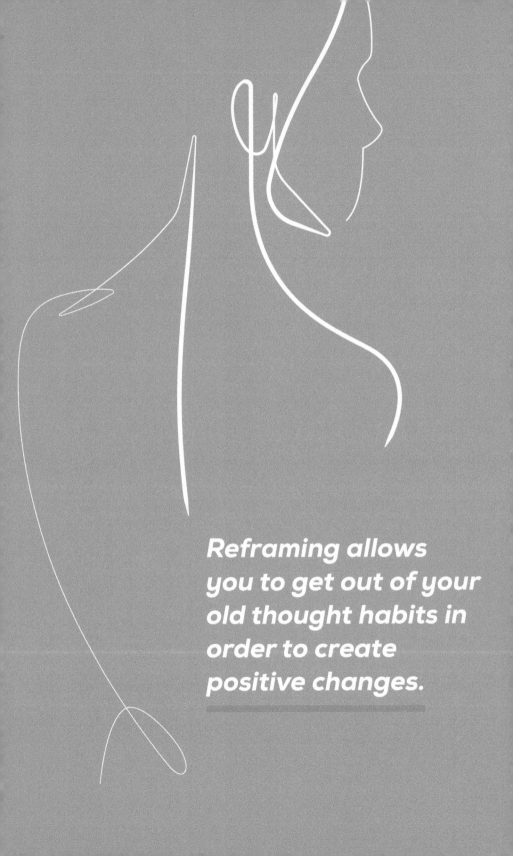

Reframing allows you to get out of your old thought habits in order to create positive changes.

CHAPTER TWO
A New Mindset

Retraining the brain requires an awareness of thoughts and habits. This chapter will look at reframing pain in a more detailed way. You'll explore the process of reframing your thoughts based on research that examines how the power of words can transform your brain chemistry and help ease your pain. As you read this chapter, think about your personal pain experience and consider how you could behold your pain differently.

Meet Jill

Jill was a health care professional whose job required enormous amounts of paperwork that took up her evenings and weekends. The job didn't really bring her much happiness, the pension and benefits were excellent, but she didn't want to quit because she wanted to retire soon. Jill decided to stick it out, even though it was taking a physical and emotional toll on her body and mind.

About 18 months before her retirement, Jill's health started to decline. She began to experience pain throughout her entire body, felt completely exhausted all the time, and wasn't sleeping well, either. Jill was diagnosed with chronic fatigue syndrome; it took very little stimulus to trigger pain and fatigue to flare up because her whole system was extra sensitive to all stimulation. Late-night paperwork or bad traffic would set off Jill's physical alarm, and she'd be in dire pain and feel completely fatigued.

Jill came to me in a last-ditch effort to find relief. She had used all of her sick time but didn't think she could continue her job. Jill's goal was to feel better so she could continue working and ultimately retire with full benefits. The key to helping Jill was teaching her new skills to calm her extra-sensitive nervous system. We used a variety of reframing techniques that allowed her to nurture her body and look at what might be contributing to the stress response.

Jill quickly discovered that she was drawn to guided reframing, along with affirmations and tai chi. She began with short, clear affirmations such as "I'm safe, my body is healing, and everything is going to be okay." I recommended some recorded guided reframing for pain relief and advised her to record her own affirmations so she could listen to them when negative self-talk started up in her mind.

Initially, Jill would wake up every morning with her body shaking with fear, a pounding headache, and aching pain in every joint. But after our early sessions, she started listening to her recordings while she was in bed. She also kept a list of affirmations on her nightstand to read in the morning. Then, if she started to feel a little better, she did five minutes of tai chi before she took her shower.

It took a month before Jill developed the habit of turning to her recorded affirmations and guided reframing when she felt depressed or began thinking negatively. Within six weeks, she slowly began to feel good enough to walk her two dogs and go to church.

With her steady commitment to her self-care, Jill began recognizing how much of her stress was impacted by automatic negative self-talk. Her favorite exercise became one that recognized "ants" (automatic negative thoughts), and she was able to insert a positive thought every time a negative thought popped up. She was actually quite skilled at coming up with funny positive thoughts, and when she started using humor in our therapy sessions, I knew she was well on the road to recovery.

She tried to go back to work, but as much as she wanted to fulfill her commitment, her body rebelled. Jill learned to understand that she needed more joy in her life, rather than working at a job that was essentially killing her. Through our reframing exercises, Jill decided to pay into her pension fund so she could retire early and receive her full benefits.

Today she is happily retired and, most days, pain-free. Jill is able to look back at that time and understand that the greatest benefit was learning how to forgive herself and listen to her body. Best of all, she now instinctively can turn to her favorite affirmation whenever she needs it: "I am safe. I am loved. I am already healing."

Reframing Your Thoughts

Reframing is the ability to see a situation from a different perspective. This can be tremendously helpful in problem-solving, decision-making, and learning about yourself and your pain. The whole aim of reframing is to shift your perspective to be more empowered, while at the same time learning new skills that allow you to have control over your thoughts. When you reframe any situation, you look at it differently and change its meaning.

For example, when you reframe a picture in your camera, you can either zoom in for a close-up picture, or zoom out for something that's a little bit more distant. The idea of reframing is to use imagery, journaling, phrases, and positive affirmations to help you creatively change your beliefs. Reframing allows you to get out of your old thought habits in order to create positive changes.

Irene Tracey, a British pain neuroscientist, found that certain areas of the brain that modulated pain were different for those who experience depression and persistent pain. Her research revealed that people who develop a more positive attitude toward life—and who are able to create positive coping and stress-management skills—experienced less pain, stress, and disability than those people who maintain a negative view about their life and circumstances.

Zooming into your pain can heighten your experience, but zooming out of it to look at the bigger picture can be the difference between thriving and just existing with your pain. You need to acknowledge how and what you're feeling in order to make changes—after all, what we don't know, we can't change. Then, instead of focusing on all the ways the pain is making your life harder or even unbearable, reframing helps you acknowledge that pain but focus on all the positive ways you are healing.

Your Thought Habits

The key to changing your thought habits is to understand that you actually have a routine of these thoughts. Habits are generally unconscious behaviors that go on in the background of our lives without too much input from our conscious minds. For example, you might get a lower back X-ray that says you have moderate degeneration, so immediately you think you need surgery. Or you notice that your knuckles are starting to swell and think that you've got rheumatoid arthritis. And of course that pain in your right shoulder is lung cancer. These are all thoughts that aren't based in reality, yet they can actually create pain.

Pain is just one protective action that the body can take. For example, when people have a heart attack, they often have pain in their arm. But there's no damage to the arm—the pain is actually coming from the heart.

Or imagine taking a big bite of a ripe, juicy lemon. Are you salivating? This is the biological response to an imaginary thought, and shows you that we can think our way into changing our body.

The example of the lemon is from Elmer Green, Ph.D., a pioneer in the world of biofeedback. He is a firm believer that people have the power to find pain relief by using the power of their minds. For example, you could change the thought "I can't go for a walk because my hip will throb" to "It's a beautiful day, and even if my hip throbs, I will enjoy walking today." It's often helpful to have a statement that you can use when you're having a pain experience. In Jill's case, her favorite affirmation allowed her to immediately feel less stressed and to zoom her perspective out instead of focusing on her pain.

Revised Thinking

Once you deconstruct your thoughts, new thought habits must be put in place. Studies on positive affirmations have been shown, through functional magnetic resonance imaging (fMRI), to be powerful changemakers in the parts of the brain responsible for executive function. These affirmations also create neurochemicals that attach to dopamine, oxytocin, and serotonin receptors in the brain.

Examples of these phenomena are athletes who train with imagery over and over before they compete in a sporting event. The beautiful thing about imagery is that the brain believes what you tell it. By revising the information that goes into your brain, you're able to change the output. For athletes, this imagery, or revised thinking, is usually about performing at their best during a competition. But it can also be applied to your pain. The brain is always scanning 360 degrees, 24 hours a day, seven days a week, to see what sort of danger you might get into. If you tell the brain that it's going to be okay, the pain you experience can often diminish.

Words are powerful. Imagine getting your MRI back and your surgeon tells you that your spinal discs have some wrinkles from aging. And since the wrinkles on your face don't hurt, most of the time wrinkles in your spine are also nonpainful. Now, compare that to a doctor saying words such as *slipped disc, ruptured, bone-on-bone,* and *degeneration.* Sounds catastrophic and serious, right?

That's not to say these issues aren't serious, but it does make you wonder about word choice and phrasing. The brain pays attention because it's looking for a threat in order to protect your body. We know from our scientific research that positive thoughts create healing chemicals in the brain. Phrases such as *hurt doesn't equal harm, motion is lotion, sore but safe, tissues heal,* and *just breathe* allow the brain to send out chemicals that help calm your pain and settle your nervous system.

Reframing Exercises

Now it's time to put your reframing techniques into practice. The following exercises start off easy and become more complex as you work through them. Remember to take your time. This may all be new to you, so no one expects you to have your practice down pat or to be perfect in your first go-around. Please practice patience with yourself. I also strongly encourage you to record yourself while completing these exercises—where it warrants—so you can have them readily available in a moment's notice.

Cultivate an Attitude of Gratitude

Good for: chronic pain, releasing tension, stress relief

When you're feeling depressed, coupled with pain and negative feelings, you may find it difficult to see the positive aspects of life. This reframing exercise consists of writing down three things that you are thankful for to create a gratitude list. The act of writing helps you organize your thoughts and become aware of how powerful your beliefs and emotions can be. This is a wonderful tool to use before bed to create new associations in your brain that focus on the positive aspects of your life. Keep it simple and honest, and don't stress about doing it every day.

Let's begin.

- Decide where you want to create your list—it could be on your computer or phone, or in a separate notebook that you keep by your bed.

- Make a list of three things that you feel gratitude for. It can be as simple as making it through the day, having a place to rest your body, or the loving presence of your pet. For example:

1. I'm grateful that my cat loves to sit on my lap.

2. I'm grateful that Prince recorded a lot of music that I can enjoy.

3. I'm grateful that I have a wonderful bed to sleep in tonight.

Remember that there is no right or wrong way to do this exercise. You don't need to buy a fancy journal. The important thing is to establish the habit of paying attention to events that can inspire gratitude in your daily life.

Reframe Your Pain Thermometer

Good for: headaches, joint pain, nerve pain,
releasing tension, stress relief

This exercise allows you to change your perception of pain in a way that doesn't involve your normal, thinking mind. You will use the imagery of a thermometer that measures your pain as a way to reframe how you think about your body. Over time, this simple exercise can be used to reduce your pain at a moment's notice. By being aware of the changes in your body, you allow your brain to revise your thought habits about pain. You will need a pen and paper to jot down some information about how you feel before and after the session.

Let's begin.

- Start by lying down or sitting on a bed, couch, or chair.

- Imagine that a digital thermometer represents the heat of your pain, from 0 to 100 degrees—0 is no pain, and 100 is scorching pain.

- Now, without overthinking this question, what number would you see on the screen of the thermometer as you rate your level of pain right now?

- Keep this picture of a thermometer in your head. Imagine that you're watching the numbers move on the screen, and the thermometer stops at the number you chose. For example, if your pain number was 85, that's the number you'd see.

- Close your eyes and imagine the number dropping down 5 degrees, as you cool down your pain.

- Then imagine it dropping down another 5 degrees.

- Continue cooling down your pain by 5 or 10 degrees at a time.

- When you feel that the number has stopped falling, take a slow and easy breath, and write down that number and a brief description of how you feel.

Timer for Change

Good for: chronic pain, joint pain, releasing tension, stress relief

In order to create ways of thinking, we have to do the work to create a habit. An easy way to accomplish this is to set a timer for every two hours throughout the day to remind you to do a particular activity. An important part of managing pain is remembering to breathe, relax your shoulders, and stop the negative self-talk. Setting a timer allows you to create habitual patterns for those.

Let's begin.

- Set a timer on your phone or watch for every two hours. Pick a tone that is pleasant or fun to hear. (My favorite is the "boing" timer because it makes me laugh.)

- Each time the alarm goes off, ask yourself three questions:

1. *What's happening to my breath?* Are you holding your breath? Is your breathing shallow?

2. *Where is my mind?* Notice what you're thinking about. Is it positive or negative?

3. *Where's my body?* How is your posture? Are you clenching your jaw? Are you holding your muscles tight? Where is your pain? Do you even have any pain at this moment?

- Moving forward, each time the alarm goes off, stop what you're doing and notice these three items. Don't look for pain, stress, or negativity. Just notice your breath, mind, and body. The brain begins to rewire its thoughts as you notice things about yourself—it's a bit like an autocorrect program.

- The more you notice that things are out of sync, the better you get at guiding yourself into a better pattern of breathing, thinking, and moving.

- I'm suggesting three important questions, but don't let that suggestion limit your imagination. It generally takes six weeks to create the neural plasticity of habituation.

- There's been some research to suggest that adding a fun element to your training accelerates this time period.
  As I mentioned before, I use the silly sound on my iPhone that makes me laugh, which creates serotonin, oxytocin, and dopamine. Who wouldn't want that nice boost of chemicals every time they try to create a good habit?

Shining a Positive Light

Good for: chronic pain, headaches, joint pain, nerve pain, stress relief

Joan Borysenko, an inspirational author, wrote about "awfulizing"—focusing on the worst possible outcomes. We all awfulize things and Google helps us get there. (Have you ever noticed that cancer pops up with just about any symptom that you write in the search box?) Our stressful thoughts only make our pain worse. But one way to change negative thoughts is through reframing them with humor or helpful answers. This involves writing down the stressful event and then trying to see it differently, in a positive light.

Let's begin.

- Start with a 9-by-11-inch piece of paper, folded in half to create a crease, but keep it unfolded.

- On the left side, make 10 to 15 lines. Here you'll write down your terrible pain stories and obsessive worry.

- On the right side, write down a realistic explanation for each, as if you were trying to calm down a nervous friend.

For example:

1. On the left: *My hip is bone-on-bone. I'm going to have to stop walking and I'm going to gain 50 pounds.*

2. On the right: *My friend had her hip replaced and now she's hiking around Europe.* Or *I have heard that hip replacements are easy now, and that might get rid of my pain.*

In this case, you're basically playing the role of your own reassuring friend, helping yourself turn your awfulizing into positive thinking. Try this out a few times each week for at least four weeks. At the end of the month, notice if your thought patterns have changed.

The Pain Interview

Good for: chronic pain, headaches, joint pain, nerve pain, stress relief

This exercise is designed as an interview with your pain. In order to change your thoughts and perceptions about pain, it's essential to learn the nitty-gritty of what's truly happening within your body.

There's a saying that where the mind goes, the energy flows. If your mind goes to negativity, frustration, and stress, that's exactly where your energy will go. It's important to identify which parts of your mind and body are involved with your pain. With this exercise, you will be able to identify your thoughts, feelings, and beliefs, which will help you look at how pain impacts your body in real time. When you begin to identify all the things that are happening during a pain episode, you begin to demystify the whole process of pain. Once you've done this several times, you may find that it's easier to do it in the moment of a pain experience.

The process of writing down what's happening in your body interrupts the unconscious pattern. It brings to light new information, and brings the possibilities of change and hope into your life at the moment that you are experiencing pain.

Let's begin.

- Find a comfortable seated position and have your notebook and pencil or pen ready.

- One at a time, write the following five questions down, stopping to think about each one and noting your response to each:

1. *What am I thinking right now?* For example, if you walk today, will it make your hip hurt more? Does it matter?

CONTINUED

2. *What am I feeling?* Make sure that you just observe what you're feeling rather than judging or changing it. The act of observing emotions and beliefs allows for change to occur. Can you think of a more positive emotion, such as gratitude for having good shoes to walk in, or relief that the sun is shining? Choose several feelings that are positive.

3. *What do I believe about this pain that I'm feeling?* Make sure that you look at whether it is true and whether you're willing to die on the sword of this particular belief. Ask yourself what happens if this is a false belief.

4. *What's going on in my body?* Bring your awareness to your body and neutrally observe where you might be holding tension. Are your knees locked? Are you tensing your jaw? Draw a picture of your body and color in the areas that you've noticed.

5. *Where is my breath?* Are you holding your breath? Is it short and rapid? Can you change your breath? Observe what happens in your body when you change your breath. Write down the changes.

Reading an interview with someone helps you understand them better, and it's the same with your pain. Once you begin to understand how it impacts your mind and body, you can then try to reframe it more positively.

Increase Your Stress Awareness

Good for: chronic pain, releasing tension, stress relief

There is no definitive survey to determine if you are stressed or burnt out. But questionnaires do help increase awareness that, indeed, there may be a problem in one or more areas of your life. The following is an example of a simple inventory to help you determine the level of stress in your life.

Let's begin.

- Read each statement and then circle either *Agree* or *Disagree*.

- Count the number of "Agree" points (one per question).

- Use the stress level key to determine your personal stress level.

1.	I have a hard time falling asleep at night.	AGREE	DISAGREE
2.	I tend to suffer from tension and/or migraine headaches.	AGREE	DISAGREE
3.	I find myself thinking about finances and making ends meet.	AGREE	DISAGREE
4.	I wish I could find more to laugh and smile about each day.	AGREE	DISAGREE
5.	More often than not, I skip breakfast or lunch to get things done.	AGREE	DISAGREE
6.	If I could change my job situation, I would.	AGREE	DISAGREE
7.	I wish I had more personal time for leisure pursuits.	AGREE	DISAGREE

CONTINUED

8.	I have lost a good friend or family member recently.	AGREE	DISAGREE
9.	I am unhappy in my relationship or am recently divorced.	AGREE	DISAGREE
10.	I haven't had a quality vacation in a long time.	AGREE	DISAGREE
11.	I wish that my life had a clear meaning and purpose.	AGREE	DISAGREE
12.	I tend to eat more than three meals a week outside the home.	AGREE	DISAGREE
13.	I tend to suffer from chronic pain.	AGREE	DISAGREE
14.	I don't have a strong group of friends to whom I can turn.	AGREE	DISAGREE
15.	I don't exercise regularly (fewer than three times per week).	AGREE	DISAGREE
16.	I am on prescribed medication for depression.	AGREE	DISAGREE
17.	My sex life is not very satisfying.	AGREE	DISAGREE
18.	My family relationships are less than desirable.	AGREE	DISAGREE
19.	Overall, my self-esteem can be rather low.	AGREE	DISAGREE
20.	I spend no time each day dedicated to meditation or centering.	AGREE	DISAGREE

Stress Level Key

Less than 5 points	You have a low level of personal stress.
More than 5 points	You have a moderate level of personal stress.
More than 10 points	You have a high level of personal stress.
More than 15 points	You have an exceptionally high level of personal stress.

This questionnaire was developed by Brian Luke Seaward, Ph.D.

Once you've determined your level of stress and the things that are causing it, you can start to address them individually and change your habits so that you can gradually work toward achieving a calmer state.

Finding Your Happy Place

Good for: chronic pain, headaches, joint pain, nerve pain, releasing tension, stress relief

People experiencing persistent pain often find that happiness seems elusive. This exercise invites you to explore what happiness means to you, and to find small things that may show you that happiness can be within your reach. Happiness is not always about things and places— for many, it's an inward journey. At its foundation, it includes a sense of stability and security in one's environment. There are many words for happiness, including contentment, inner peace, joy, love, and bliss. And while there is no magic formula or road map to follow, happiness is within everyone's reach.

Pam Grout, the author of *E-Squared*, writes about manifesting anything that you want by imagining it and expecting it to be so. The process of dreaming into your life and envisioning what you want has been shown to be a powerful spiritual exercise with endless possibilities. If your pain keeps you from canoeing or hiking, find pictures of hikers and people enjoying water sports. In order to change your perception of what you can do in your life and how much happiness you are able to enjoy, you must understand what that concept actually means to you. In this exercise, you will make a picture board to help you manifest your dreams.

Let's begin.

- Set up a workspace with paper, pencils, glue, magazines, and photos (optional).

- While you ask yourself each of the following questions, draw or find pictures that represent things that might bring happiness into your life.

1. What does the concept of "happiness" mean to you?

2. Would you call yourself a happy person? Why or why not?

3. Why do you think there is such a drive to find happiness in American culture? Could stress have something to do with this?

4. What would you say are some obvious roadblocks to happiness? List as many as you can.

5. Where is your happy place? Where do you go to find or, better yet, surround yourself with happiness? Where do you surround yourself in beauty?

6. How does your sense of humor play into your sense of happiness?

7. Any other thoughts about happiness?

Use this space to make a personal strategy for creating happiness. Think about the activities you can do, the behaviors you can adopt, the places you can go, and the dreams you can manifest. What intentions can you birth to reinforce the ideals of bringing a sense of balance into your life through the front door of happiness?

This exercise was influenced by Brian Luke Seaward, Ph.D.

Self-Healing through Tapping and Affirmations

Good for: headaches, nerve pain, releasing tension, stress relief

Dr. Daniel J. Benor created a technique known as Transformative Wholistic Reintegration (TWR), which combines a practice known as tapping with eye movement desensitization and reprocessing (EMDR). He developed it in order to create a self-healing tool that is accessible, easy to perform, and effective for pain and healing.

TWR is a simple practice involving four steps: identify the thought or feeling, tap it out, assess how you feel, and then reframe a new thought or feeling. It's helpful to write down your thoughts and feelings in a journal because they will change throughout this process.

Once you've learned the steps, you can successfully do this in your car, in a grocery line, or at your desk. Work on your issues when you're not stressed, so you get the hang of it.

Let's begin.

- Identify a feeling, thought, or pain sensation that you would like to change. How strong is it on a scale from 0 (it doesn't bother you at all) to 10 (the worst you could possibly feel)? This is called the Subjective Units of Distress Scale (SUDS).

- Next, stimulate the right and left sides of the body by doing one of the following:

1. Move your eyes back and forth from right to left.

2. While sitting down, tap the right and left eyebrows with one hand at the point nearest the nose.

3. Pat the biceps of each arm (arms crossed so that the right hand taps left bicep, and vice versa).

4. Tap your feet right and left while you're standing or sitting.

- While you are doing your right/left tapping, say a positive affirmation such as those that follow. Most people will find that this is an effective way of reducing the negative feelings and thoughts. After tapping for a few more minutes, check the SUDS again—it will usually go down. Repeat the assessing and tapping until the SUDS is zero.

1. "Even though I have this [pain, anxiety, panic, fear], I love and accept myself unconditionally, and [God/Christ/Allah/ the Infinite Source] loves and accepts me completely and unconditionally."

2. "Even though I'm afraid that my hip pain will keep me awake all night, I love myself unconditionally, and [God/ Christ/Allah/the Infinite Source] loves me completely and unconditionally."

3. Any other strong positive affirmation that feels good for you.

- Next, add your replacement positive affirmation that counters the negative one that's been released. For example:

1. "I'm comfortable [looking down from any height/thinking about being near spiders/whatever your issue is]. I love and accept myself unconditionally, and [God/Christ/Allah/the Infinite Source] loves and accepts me unconditionally."

CONTINUED

2. "Even though my hip hurts, I expect and deserve sleep that's fully restorative. I love and accept myself unconditionally, and [God/Christ/Allah/the Infinite Source] accepts me unconditionally."

While the procedures for doing TWR are simple, the releasing of symptoms and problems may be complicated. For instance, if the number is not moving (down when dealing with the problem or up when installing the replacement affirmation), we can identify the issues that are blocking progress. In fact, blocks may be very helpful clues to deeper beliefs that keep us stuck in the ruts and vicious circles we have created in our lives.

Used with permission from Daniel J. Benor, M.D., DanielBenor.com.

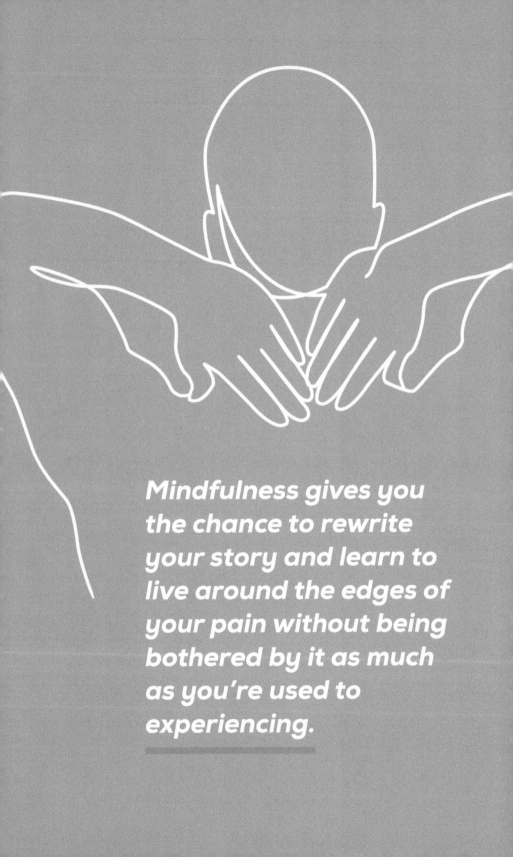

Mindfulness gives you the chance to rewrite your story and learn to live around the edges of your pain without being bothered by it as much as you're used to experiencing.

CHAPTER THREE

Stay in the Present

Jon Kabat-Zinn describes mindfulness as "paying attention to something in a particular way, on purpose, in the present moment, non-judgmentally." This chapter is about mindfulness in the context of using it for pain relief, and learning how to move into your pain with curiosity and courage.

Meet Emily

Emily was referred to me in order to learn self-regulation exercises to help with her headaches and fibromyalgia. From the start, she believed that no matter what type of exercise she did, her pain would always return.

Emily was almost proud that nobody could make her pain go away; she wore her pain like a badge of honor, even though at 32 years old, she was working on getting disability benefits.

She moved slowly and was nervous about starting any sort of program that might make her pain worse. I promised to go nice and easy and that she was in charge of the session and could stop anytime she needed. I knew that many of the rehab exercises had not been successful, and though her medications numbed the pain, they never took it away fully. When I asked Emily where she hurt, her answer was "everywhere." This is common in people with fibromyalgia or chronic fatigue syndrome.

Mindfulness techniques seemed to be a good place for Emily to start. Her history was typical for somebody with chronic pain. She had experienced childhood abuse and many unsuccessful interventions, as well as being told that her pain was all in her head and not real. She explained to me how the pain could start in her foot, move all the way up her leg and into her back, and grab onto her neck.

As she described her pain, I pulled out a picture of a body that had been donated to science for research on nerves. Researchers were surprised to discover that all of the nerves were connected, from the toes to the head. It made sense to me that her foot pain could move all the way up to her neck.

We began our first session with pain neuroscience education. I explained that we have an equal distribution of chemical channels in our nerves, sort of like doors that open and help the brain know what's happening to the body. They provide information about pain, stress, temperature, movement, and blood flow. When your brain thinks you are under threat, like from a sudden or chronic pain, the body makes more pain channels. If you have to drive in a congested rush hour every day, you may create more stress channels. If you have the flu, you get more chemical inflammation channels, resulting in more pain. Once you begin exercises to calm the brain and reduce pain, the "threat" leaves, and the channel distributions rebalance. One of the beauties of mindfulness is its simplicity.

Emily and I did a body scan and a visualization exercise that allowed her to notice a painful area and then release the pain. Each time we released one region, she would excitedly say, "Now this region hurts!" We talked about the communication of the nervous system, how the squeaky wheel—or loudest pain—gets noticed, and why pain can be experienced in the whole system because of its connectivity. We continued with awareness and releasing, and after 55 minutes, she finally had complete relaxation.

The most important part of this exercise was to have Emily notice the change that happened in her body once she released the pain. This has to do with the habit of the brain not caring whether you have pain. In order to make the changes stick, you have to be aware that the pain is there and that change has occurred. If she had looked for her pain after doing this one-hour exercise, she would have found it, because she had the habit of feeling pain throughout her whole body.

Now she had tools that she knew could release her pain. We know that where the mind goes, the energy flows, so Emily allowed her mind to be placed in a state of rest, with an expectation that she would feel better. It took her four weeks to master this skill of going into her pain, releasing it, and not looking for it when she was done.

What Is Mindfulness?

Mindfulness is a state of being rather than an action. It directs your attention to the present moment. It's about paying attention to *how* you pay attention. Chronic pain is one of the most common symptoms to drive people to join a mindfulness class. Many of the participants have tried almost every medical intervention, and they come to mindfulness thinking that it might make the pain go away.

What mindfulness does is tap into the body's natural ability to calm itself and reduce pain. A 2011 study in the *Journal of Neuroscience* showed that mindfulness practices reduced pain unpleasantness by 57 percent and reduced pain intensity by 40 percent. Mindfulness can be used for most types of pain, including neuropathic pain. Research has shown that mindfulness also reduces the stress-related components of unrelenting pain, and it can be used as a companion to appropriate medications.

Most people who experience chronic pain tend to distract their attention away from painful sensations. This is understandable, because the mind sees pain as something that is undesirable and therefore should be pushed away. But pushing pain away is exhausting and can use up the brain's natural calming chemicals.

Mindfulness techniques teach you how to relate differently to your experiences, including pain. I can say with conviction that the practice can help you develop the ability to cope better and feel more moments of joy—while still being aware of the pain. Mindfulness gives you the chance to rewrite your story and learn to live around the edges of your pain without being bothered by it as much as you're used to experiencing.

Curiosity Required

Mindfulness without curiosity is impossible. When we're on our day-to-day autopilot, we don't notice things. Have you ever heard the song of a bird and stopped to listen, only to begin to notice that there are more birds? I've got news for you—those birds were there the whole time, yet you didn't hear them because you had not yet stopped to listen. Mindfulness requires the act of looking at something with different eyes. It changes our perception of the moment and allows us to be curious about what might be happening inside our body that creates pain.

With mindfulness, we want to observe our experience as it takes place—including any pain that might be present. When you add mindfulness as a tool to treat your pain, you're being asked to notice things such as tingling, pulsing, throbbing, heat, cold, aching, tightness, and so on. When you let go of the pain label, you start noticing the things about pain and the sensations that accompany it. When you see pain through curious eyes, it allows you to let go of the battle of escaping or avoiding it, or of looking at it from outside the body.

The act of noticing something is very different from looking at something. For example, look at the wall in front of you. Now, take a moment to feel what is happening in your body. This is an action that has an energy to it. Now, notice the wall in front of you, allowing the color, the shape, and any objects on the wall to come into your focus. Did that feel different than looking? Noticing is quiet and inwardly focused. Mindfulness allows us to be in the moment without any agenda.

When you're experiencing pain, you may often have a thought about that pain and what's causing it. If you were to just notice the pain—without the other stories—how is that different for you? You've basically taken away the stories about your pain and allowed yourself to be present with what's there.

Focused Attention

Mindfulness practice isn't about shutting out the pain. It's about leaning into the pain and learning about the nuances that it might present. Rather than making just a blanket statement, such as "I have pain all the time," take the time to be curious. By focusing your attention on the quality and timing of your pain, you can start to understand yourself more fully. The act of noticing your pain and being present for your whole body will transform your relationship with pain.

We often have expectations about experiences that might increase or alleviate pain, which may or may not be true. As human beings, we tend to be habit makers, and these habits create an unconscious groove into which we fall without any thought. By moving into a quieter and kinder relationship with your pain, you may discover that your pain isn't present all the time, or that having cookies makes your pain worse while coloring in a book reduces your pain. You begin to create a new habit of noticing. You can't know what changes the quality and the intensity of your pain if you don't pay attention to it. Anyone with chronic pain knows that it's easy to put everything in the basket of "My whole body hurts; therefore, I have to be really careful."

Mindfulness allows you to tease out the different facets of your pain and feelings. It quietly allows you to take a peek inside yourself, without any judgment, for a short period of time. You may be surprised by what happens when you focus your attention on a regular basis.

Mindfulness Exercises

I recommend that you record the following exercises using an app on your phone if possible. Hearing your own voice guiding you into a visualization or body scan tends to have a very affirming effect on your behavior. Telling yourself how to relax and what to do is a very powerful way to listen to visualizations. When your body is in pain, it's very difficult to initiate a relaxation exercise because of the interruptions and the inability to stay focused and present. By using guided visualizations, you can learn to relax your body and calm your busy mind.

Five Senses Exercise

When you feel stress or anxiety, due to pain or another reason, it's often hard to stay grounded and present. This exercise helps you to shift your focus to your surroundings in the present moment, and away from what is causing you to feel anxious, while interrupting unhealthy thought patterns.

The goal of this exercise is to practice being aware in the present moment throughout the day, whenever formal mindfulness practice such as meditation or a body scan might not be practical. All that is needed is to notice something you are experiencing with each of the five senses.

Let's begin.

- Notice five things that you can see. Look around you and bring your attention to five things that you can see. Pick things that you don't normally notice, like a shadow, a small crack in the concrete, or a spot on the ceiling.

- Notice four things that you can feel. Bring awareness to four things that you are currently feeling, like the texture of your pants, the feel of your hair, or the sensation of a ring on your finger.

- Notice three things you can hear. Take a moment to listen, and note three things that you hear in the background. This can be the chirp of a bird, the hum of the refrigerator, or the faint sound of traffic from a nearby road.

CONTINUED

- Notice two things you can smell. Bring your awareness to smells that you usually filter out, whether they're pleasant or unpleasant. If you're in your office, you can smell your pencil or notice the smell of soap on your skin. If you're outside, notice the smell of a fast-food restaurant or the smell of exhaust from cars as they drive by.

- Notice one thing you can taste. Focus on one thing that you can taste right now, at this moment. Notice the taste in your mouth, take a sip of a drink if you have it near you, or even taste the salt on your skin on your upper lip.

Five-Minute Guided Meditation for Pain

Good for: chronic pain, headaches, joint pain, releasing tension, stress relief

This easy-to-follow meditation serves as an introduction to pain management. If you need to make minor modifications to accommodate your pain, feel free to do so without guilt. The goal is comfort, not discomfort.

Let's begin.

- Get into whatever position is most comfortable for you with the pain you are currently experiencing.

- Gently close your eyes. If possible, place your hands on your pain. If not, just let your hands rest comfortably.

- Take a long, deep inhale through your nose, allowing your breath to expand fully, and hold your breath at the top. When you're ready, exhale with a sigh.

- At the end of that breath, return to a pattern of breathing that feels right for you.

- Breathe in through your nose and out through your mouth throughout this meditation. Ensure that your stomach is expanding on every inhale and contracting on every exhale. Feel yourself enter into a flow with this breathing pattern.

- While you stay focused on your breath, additionally allow your awareness to center on the pain you are experiencing. Allow yourself to really feel it.

- As you let yourself feel whatever is coming over you as it relates to this pain, allow yourself to imagine your breath flowing into this area of your body.

CONTINUED

- Notice yourself shifting away from all of the frustration and all of the emotions that you were just experiencing, and instead notice how you are entering into a place of acceptance. Accept your pain with love—not asking it to leave, just sending it healing energy and loving acceptance.

- As you listen to the message your pain has for you, accepting it with love, you may notice that it actually begins to soften. In this moment, you are actually getting to the root of the pain.

- Spend as much time as you need to breathe into the area where you are experiencing pain.

- Do this as long as you need to, and when you are ready, very slowly and gently bring your awareness back to the room around you.

- Open your eyes when it feels right to you.

Breathing into your pain allows you to acknowledge it rather than pushing it away. By accepting it with love, you can slowly begin to heal it.

15-Minute Body Scan

Good for: chronic pain, headaches, joint pain, nerve pain, releasing tension

This body scan can be done while lying down, sitting, or in any other posture. It's truly an exercise about developing awareness. The steps are a guided meditation. Once you've done it several times while reading the instructions (or having them read back to you), it's easy to do at night if you find that you have trouble either initiating sleep or returning to sleep after waking up. This helps you become aware of how you feel when your muscles are tense, and how you feel when they are relaxed. With practice, you can easily notice tension and quickly relax.

Let's begin.

- Start by bringing your attention into your body

- You can close your eyes if it's comfortable for you.

- Notice the weight of your body, whether it's in a chair, on a couch, or on the floor.

- Take a few deep breaths.

- As you take a deeper breath, bring in more oxygen and feel it filling the cells of your body. As you exhale, focus on a sense of relaxing more deeply.

- Notice the sensations of your feet, wherever they may be. Feel the weight, pressure, vibration, and heat.

- Notice your legs and feel the pressure, pulsing, heaviness, and lightness.

- Notice your spine. Feel the weight of it in your back.

- Bring your attention to your stomach area. If your stomach is tense, let it soften. Take a breath.

CONTINUED

- Notice if your hands feel tight. See if you can allow them to soften.

- Feel any sensation in your arms. Let your shoulders be soft.

- Notice your neck and throat. Let them be soft. Relax.

- Soften your jaw. Let your face and facial muscles soften.

- Notice how your whole body is present. Take a deep breath. Notice how your body feels when you are feeling it with breath.

- Be aware of your whole body as best you can. Take a breath. When you're ready, slowly blink your eyes open.

This exercise is best done three times a week for anywhere between 10 and 20 minutes.

Progressive Muscle Relaxation Script

Good for: chronic pain, headaches, joint pain,
releasing tension, stress relief

This exercise reduces stress and anxiety in your body by having you slowly tense and then relax each muscle. You can use it to provide an immediate feeling of relaxation, but it's best to do it frequently. With practice, you will become more aware of when you are experiencing tension, and you will have the skills to help you relax. During this exercise, each muscle should be tensed, but not to the point of strain. If you have any injuries or pain, you can skip the affected areas. Pay special attention to the feeling of releasing tension in each muscle and the resulting feeling of relaxation.

Let's begin.

- Begin by taking a deep breath and noticing the feeling of air filling your lungs. Hold your breath for a few seconds. Pause briefly; then release the breath slowly while letting the tension leave your body.

- Take another deep breath and hold it. Again, slowly release the air.

- Even more slowly, take another breath. Fill your lungs and hold the breath; then gradually release it and imagine the feeling of tension leaving your body.

- Now, move your attention to your feet. Begin to tense your feet by curling your toes toward the arch of your foot. Hold onto the tension and notice what it feels like.

- Release the tension in your toes and feel the sense of relaxation.

CONTINUED

Progressive Muscle Relaxation
Script *CONTINUED*

- Next, begin to focus on your lower leg. Tense the muscles in your calves, hold them tightly, and pay attention to the feeling of tension.

- Release the tension from your lower legs. Again, notice the feeling of relaxation. Remember to continue taking slow, easy breaths.

- Next, tense the muscles of your upper legs and pelvis. You can do this by lightly squeezing your thighs together. Make sure you feel the tenseness without going to the point of strain.

- Now release. Feel the tension leave your muscles.

- Begin to tense your stomach and chest by sucking your stomach in. Squeeze harder and hold the tension. If it hurts, just *imagine* that you're holding this tension, rather than doing it physically. Your brain won't know the difference.

- Release the tension. Allow your body to go limp. Let yourself notice the feeling of relaxation.

- Continue taking deep breaths. Breathe slowly, noticing the air filling your lungs, and hold it. Release the air slowly, feeling it leave your lungs.

- Next, tense the muscles in your back by bringing your shoulders together behind you. Hold them tightly. Tense them as hard as you can without straining, and keep holding them.

- Release the tension from your back. Feel the tension slowly leaving your body in the new feeling of relaxation. Notice how different your body feels when you allow it to relax.

- Tense your arms all the way up from your hands to your shoulders. Make a fist and squeeze all the way up your arms.

- Release the tension from your arms and shoulders. Notice the feeling of relaxation in your fingers, hands, arms, and shoulders. Notice how your arms feel limp and at ease.

- Move up your neck to your head. Tense your face and scrunch your face muscles and squeeze your eyes tightly.

- Release the tension. Again, notice the new feelings of relaxation.

- Finally, tense your entire body— your feet, legs, stomach, chest, arms, head, and neck. Tense harder, without straining. Hold the tension.

- Now release. Allow your whole body to go limp. Pay attention to the feeling of relaxation, and notice how different it is from the feeling of tension.

- As you begin to slowly wake up your body by moving your muscles, gently roll your neck around, adjust your arms and legs, and blink your eyes open. Notice how your body feels, and take a deep breath, allowing yourself to feel the ease in support of your body.

Mindful Emotions

Good for: chronic pain, headaches, nerve pain, releasing tension, stress relief

We all experience a steady stream of emotions throughout the day. Often these emotions coincide with a pain experience, but all too often we discount it. This exercise will help you tune into your emotions, your judgments about them, and their ebb and flow as you're feeling them. Part of forming a healthy, healing relationship with your emotions is allowing yourself to acknowledge them.

Whenever you feel the need to process emotions or understand why you are feeling a certain way, you can use this exercise. You can either write down your feelings or—if you want to use this more as a mindfulness awareness technique—just notice your body as you read each question. Try this exercise in the morning and the evening to see which time of day is best suited for you.

Let's begin.

- Take a few moments to focus on your breathing. Notice your breathing without changing it.

- Notice how you feel emotionally in the present moment. Without judging, just be aware of how you feel.

- What emotion are you experiencing? Name the emotion.

- Is it pleasant or unpleasant? Notice if it feels good or not good.

- Is the feeling steady or coming and going?

- Is it changing in intensity? How is it changing?

- Gently maintain your attention on your emotion.

- Have you felt this emotion before? Is it coming from the past or the present?

- What is the present moment of the emotion?

- How are you breathing?

- How does your posture match the feeling?

- How does the emotion show up in your body?

- Is there any part of your body that is uncomfortable? Have you noticed this body sensation before?

- Are your muscles tense or relaxed?

- What is your facial expression?

- As you notice thoughts, simply acknowledge them, dismiss them, and bring your attention back to your emotion.

- Allow and accept instead of judging.

- As one emotion subsides and another emotion arises, simply repeat the process.

Mindful Noticing

Good for: chronic pain, stress relief

When we look at things, we're making sense of objects, textures, and sounds all at once. The act of noticing requires you to be present with all of your senses. With this exercise, you will be asked to notice your surroundings without making a story, adding commentary, or judging what you see. This is a simple exercise that you could scale from 10 to 20 minutes, and requires a window or being outdoors. There is no need for any notebook or pen unless you would like to make notes after the exercise.

Each time you find your mind wandering and pull it back to a calm, undistracted place, you are creating neural pathways in your brain. This is how you create new, healthy habits. Make sure to notice when you stray from this process and bring yourself back to your place of breath and peace. Becoming aware of your mindful behavior allows you to create a sustainable change.

Let's begin.

- Find your comfortable sitting or standing position, either indoors or outdoors, where there are sights to see.

- Start by practicing feeling the difference between noticing something and seeing something. Look at an object with your eyes intently. Feel what happens to your body, face, and eyes as you are looking.

- Now allow the object you were looking at to come into your view and be noticed, rather than directly focused on. This is a passive experience. Feel what happens to your body, breath, and eyes. Many people will feel a softening relaxation effect.

- Stop and pause.

- Now, with soft, noticing eyes, look around at everything there is to see. Avoid labeling and categorizing what you see. For example, instead of thinking "bird" or "stop sign," try to notice the colors, patterns, and textures of those things.

- Pay attention to the movement of the grass or leaves in the breeze. Notice the many different shapes present in the small segment of the world that you can see. Try to see the world from the perspective of someone seeing it for the first time.

- Be observant but not critical. Be aware but not fixated.

- If you become distracted and find yourself thinking, comparing, or judging, gently pull your mind away from those thoughts and notice a color or shape again to put you back in the right frame of mind.

- Notice how your body, breath, and posture feel as you end this session.

- Take note of whether your mind was busy, or whether you were able to come back to the place of mindfully noticing.

Mindfully Calming
an Emotional Storm

Good for: headaches, nerve pain, releasing tension, stress relief

When emotions are high and life is filled with stress, a mindfulness practice is invaluable. By practicing mindfulness regularly, you can cultivate emotional stability and well-being, helping heal turmoil on a mental, emotional, and spiritual level. Because this exercise deals with your emotional health, it's important to not worry about doing it correctly or judging if you're feeling the right feelings. It's designed to provide relief from grief, pain, sorrow, and any other emotional challenges that that you may feel.

Let's begin.

- Relax into a comfortable, well-supported position, either sitting or lying down.

- Begin to breathe naturally, allowing your stomach to expand with the inhale and letting your breath spill out of you with no effort at all.

- Continue breathing and simply observe your breath coming in, filling your lungs, and falling out of you.

- Follow your breath into your body and feel it moving in and out through your tissue, bones, and nerves.

- Feel your chest and stomach expand as air flows in and contract as the air flows out.

- Become aware of the life force moving through you, filling you with renewed energy and relieving you of any stale, old, and painful energy.

- When you feel calm and comfortable, slowly allow your body to relax.

- Gently bring awareness to one area at a time.

- Start with your entire face, neck, and shoulders; then move down into your heart and lungs. Let your awareness move into your legs and arms as well.

- Rest in awareness here for a while; let your heart open and relax until you feel a sense of peacefulness throughout your whole being.

- Once you're relaxed, focus on your emotions. Try not to analyze or fix them. Lovingly give yourself permission to feel them exactly the way they are. Don't be afraid to experience the full force of your emotions.

- Visualize what you would like to do with these emotions. Perhaps it's screaming, kicking, or breaking things—just think about it as if you were doing it.

- Observe your emotions as they begin to release and diminish.

- As you continue to focus all your energies on this irritation or issue, you're beginning to release your negativity and emotional obstacles.

- Think of somebody you love who fully supports you. It could be somebody who has passed.

- Talk to this person about how you were just feeling either out loud or in your mind.

- Explain how and why you are feeling that way. Offer these emotions to the person as freely as you can, allowing them to take and transform them.

- When you're ready, thank this person for all they have done for you. Bless them and all the people in your life who have moved you through your challenges.

CONTINUED

Mindfully Calming an Emotional
Storm CONTINUED

* When you're ready, take several deep breaths, breathing in joy and exhaling peace.

* Continue this until you're centered and grounded with yourself once again, noticing any changes in your body, mind, and breath as you come back to your comfortable space.

Do this exercise as often as you need to. Just as a turbulent storm eventually subsides, you can learn to do the same with your mental, emotional, and spiritual turmoil.

Dissolving Pain

Good for: chronic pain, headaches, joint pain, nerve pain, releasing tension

Pain tends to demand attention. When you are experiencing pain, you tend to tighten muscles around the area, taking shallow breaths and paying very close attention to what's happening in your body. Using your breath, this exercise will bring you deep into your body—and your pain—and dissolve the pain with imagery and intent. It takes some practice to learn how to shift your attention both inward and outward, but by moving your attention consciously, you can learn to master your pain.

I have found that using this process for 10 to 15 minutes in the morning and evening can help reset the body to a neutral state of being. Often, there is cumulative physical and mental stress from either poor sleep or a long day of activity.

I would recommend practicing this process when you're not in tremendous pain in order to have small successes at the start.

Let's begin.

- Take a comfortable, deep breath and exhale.

- Feel the temperature of the air as you breathe through your nostrils, and notice the feeling in your abdomen as you exhale. Shifting your attention to your breath immediately calms your body.

- Take three comfortable and easy breaths and notice what happens in your body.

- Allow your attention to move out of your body and outside the walls of your room, outside your house, and into the yard or area surrounding your building. Notice how you feel when your attention moves broadly away from you.

CONTINUED

- Take a slow, comfortable breath and allow your attention to move back into your body. Do this several times, noticing whether it is easy or difficult.

- Allow your attention to move through the floor and into the earth. Take a deep breath and draw your attention back in your body.

- Take a slow, comfortable breath and allow your attention to move through the ceiling and up into the atmosphere. Now bring that attention back into your body.

- Notice how you feel. If thoughts come in, release them as you come back to your breath. This process is teaching you how to shift your attention with intention.

- If you have pain in your body, allow your attention to move into that area. Imagine that your attention will dissolve that pain, much like dish detergent dissolves grease.

- As you notice the area of pain, imagine that it is releasing, becoming lighter, and dissolving. If you like, you can add a color, shape, or texture to the area of pain that you are paying attention to. As you add more of your senses to this pain-dissolving technique, your body engages in this process in a more powerful way.

- Continue to breathe into and dissolve the pain until you feel it dissipate and you come to a place of ease and comfort. You may not be pain-free, but notice the quality of your breath, body, and mind.

- If you are experiencing pain in multiple regions of your body, use this exercise to wash each of them with your focused attention.

Know that you are capable of dissolving, releasing, and softening any areas of pain that exist within your body. You can do this exercise on the fly whenever you experience pain, or use it to help you find compassion and relaxation within your body.

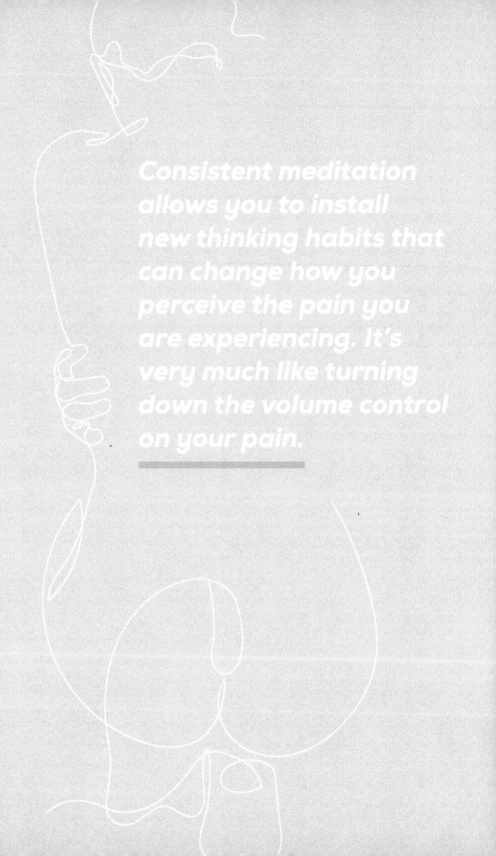

Consistent meditation allows you to install new thinking habits that can change how you perceive the pain you are experiencing. It's very much like turning down the volume control on your pain.

CHAPTER FOUR

A Deeper Connection

Meditation uses relaxation, mindfulness, and introspection to get at the root of stress and pain. In other words, to look inside yourself for pain relief, rather than external sources. This chapter invites you to go deeper into your exploration of mind-body connections to ease your pain.

Meet John

John had worked as a tool-and-die maker for over 20 years when a shelving unit unexpectedly fell on him from behind. Not only did he go into shock when the accident happened, but he lost consciousness and sustained a head injury. It was his third concussion.

Though he loved his job, John was unable to sustain the type of work that involved standing on his feet for eight hours or listening to noisy equipment. He experienced headaches, poor sleep, extreme lower back pain, and neck pain. Though he had been to physical therapy early on and improved enough to work three hours a day, his employer was pushing him to retire or find some other work. John desperately wanted to continue working in his field—it brought him joy, and many of his coworkers were his best friends.

Together John and I explored sustainable exercises and looked at what was working and what needed to change. When dealing with chronic pain, one has to be a detective—food, sleep, mood, and self-talk are all integral parts of self-care. We discussed meditation, mindfulness, and changing the story that he told himself every day about his pain. I also talked about research that shows that cumulative head injuries—like three concussions—make recovery even more difficult.

John liked to jot things down because it helped him keep track of where his thoughts were and what exercises he had done, so we used journaling to keep track of progress. He created a log for each hour of the day where he wrote down what he ate, how he felt, and what movement exercises he was doing. We also had a category for sleep, and he used a fitness tracker to make sleep tracking easier.

Since John had difficulty concentrating, we decided that we would use guided meditations, so he could listen to instructions about relaxing his body, releasing his pain, and looking more deeply at his thoughts regarding his pain, job, and general life situation. John was reluctant to use meditation for healing because of what he called his "busy brain," but he was willing to try.

I decided to use three different guided meditations—5, 20, and 60 minutes long—throughout the week. One of the meditations utilized binaural beats as part of the soundtracks to allow his brain state to go into a deeper place of relaxation. This technique helps manifest more relaxed muscles and a calmer nervous system. This is a type of biofeedback that allowed him to experience something that he couldn't normally feel in his day-to-day activities.

By discerning the difference in how he felt before the meditation, during the meditation, and after the meditation, John developed the capacity to understand what relaxed muscles truly felt like. He witnessed how meditation calmed his mind and helped him reduce some of the negative self-talk that had been part of his daily personal soundtrack. He learned how to reproduce those feelings of calm and relaxation on his own.

In six weeks, John was able to work five days a week at his job, but still needed deeper rest on the weekends. He continued to do his daily rehab exercises and found that his food choices affected his sleep, which affected his mood, which affected his pain levels. The act of writing down this information enabled John to see the integrated mind-body connection in order to change it. He recognized that if you can't see it, you can't change it.

I checked in with John one year after his last visit, and he was pleased to report that he continued to meditate three times a week, his marriage had improved, and he was back to working full-time. He said the biggest gift of his injury was learning how connected everything in his life was, and that he had improved his diet, his sleep, and, ultimately, his life.

The Basics of Meditation

The practice of meditation is thousands of years old, but the research on its health benefits is relatively new. A 2014 article in *JAMA Internal Medicine* revealed the meditation was helpful for relieving anxiety, pain, and depression. Meditation does its work through the effect of the sympathetic nervous system, which increases heart rate, breathing, and blood pressure during times of stress and pain.

I personally believe that meditation is one of the most useful and effective ways to get to a place of relaxation with almost no effort at all. But it's often a misunderstood practice. Many people proudly proclaim that their minds are just too busy to have any sort of success with meditation. We call that having a "monkey mind." I have a pretty busy brain, too, and I let it roam before doing my own meditation.

Meditation decreases activity in the brain area that's responsible for the "monkey mind." The busy brain seems to be a human problem. We are always busy sorting, deciding, and making decisions about things from the past, present, and future.

Amit Sood, professor of medicine at the Mayo Clinic, has shown that meditation creates new neural connections in the part of the brain that's responsible for monkey mind and distracted thinking. Several weeks of training can lead to improved concentration and attention, as well as reduced anxiety, pain, and stress.

Meditation is not a cure-all, but it is an important part of a mind-body connection toolkit that will allow you to change the state of your brain and, as a result, change how you think about pain, stress, and life as a whole.

A Revised Perspective

By meditating regularly, you can change how you look at certain situations in your life. Look at John. The practice enabled to him to see how depression and grief over the loss of a job that he loved was impacting his pain and stress. Pain is real—always remember that. It's the decision that the brain makes about how to respond to the body's experience that makes you have a pain experience. Meditation actually changes the wiring in your brain, building new neural pathways so that your brain will think about pain differently.

Consistent meditation allows you to install new thinking habits, which can change how you perceive the pain you are experiencing. It's very much like turning down the volume control on your pain. Pain prescriptions tend to lose their efficacy with long-term use, and there are many pain conditions that require ongoing or increased medication. But research shows that adding meditation and other self-care techniques can improve the pain condition without having to increase the medication dose.

Meditation is like physical exercise—the more you do it, the more you begin to relax, and the easier it gets. Most people have doubts and fears about meditation. Even seasoned meditators, including the Dalai Lama, often experience the monkey mind and an inability to settle thoughts. But as you continue the process of coming back to the breath, you begin to shift your thoughts and create space for change.

One of the major aims and purposes of religious practice for the individual is an inner transformation from an undisciplined, untamed, unfocused state of mind toward one that is disciplined, tamed, and balanced.

—His Holiness the Dalai Lama

Meditation Exercises

The act of recording a guided meditation and then listening to it with your own voice is a powerful way to retrain the brain. You are basically telling yourself all these amazing things—and the brain tends to believe what it's told. It allows you to reframe your thoughts and change your brain chemistry. I strongly encourage you to record yourself reciting the different exercises in this book.

Single Breath
Mantra Meditation

Good for: headaches, nerve pain, releasing tension, stress relief

While practicing meditation, you may find yourself fighting an overactive mind—planning dinner, making grocery lists, or having pretend conversations with people. To meditate deeply, it's important to quiet the mind. The more you do this, the more effective your meditation sessions will be. New brain habits take time to create, and the simpler you make these exercises, the more sustainable they become.

We will be using the Hong Sau mantra—meaning "I am spirit"—in this meditation, mentally saying the word *hong* (rhymes with *song*) as you inhale, and the word *sau* (sounds like *saw*) as you exhale.

Let's begin.

- Find a place to relax, sitting upright or supported in any position that allows you comfort.

- Close your eyes and inhale slowly, counting to eight. Hold the breath for another eight counts while concentrating your attention at the point between the eyebrows.

- Now exhale slowly to the same count of eight.

- Repeat three to six times.

- After inhaling and exhaling completely, as the next breath comes in, mentally say *hong*. And as you exhale, mentally say *sau*.

- Inhale: *hong*. Exhale: *sau*.

- Keep your eyes focused and steady at the point between your eyebrows.

- Make no attempt to control your breathing; just let it flow and be completely natural. Try to feel that your breath itself is making the sounds of the *hong* and the *sau.*

- Initially, try to feel the breath just as it enters the nostrils. Be attentive. If you have difficulty feeling the breath, you can concentrate for a while on the breathing process itself, feeling your diaphragm and chest expanding and contracting.

- Gradually, as you become calmer, try to feel the breath higher and higher in the nose. Be sure that your gaze is kept steady at the point between the eyebrows throughout the practice.

- Don't allow your eyes to follow the movement of the breath. If you find that your mind has wandered, simply bring it back to an awareness of the breath and the mantra of Hong Sau.

Mantras are useful for helping you stay focused and keeping your mind from wandering. This technique can be used anywhere from 5 minutes to, eventually, several hours.

Walking Meditation

Good for: chronic pain, joint pain, releasing tension, stress relief

A walking meditation can help you cultivate an awareness of how you feel in your body in each moment. This meditation allows you to bring your body, heart, and mind together as you move through life. Walking may be painful for you, but even at a slower pace, this meditation will help you anchor awareness of how you move your body with grace and presence. You can do this meditation as a standing meditation as well.

Let's begin.

- Choose a place either indoors or outside that is 10 to 30 paces long. If you choose to go for a longer walk, these instructions can be used for that as well.

- Start by standing still and sensing the weight of your body and your feet, feeling the muscles supporting you and stabilizing your whole bone structure. Notice how your weight feels on your right foot and then your left. Feel your legs attaching to your pelvis, and feel how your spine arises from the support of your pelvis into the neck and shoulders, which support the weight of your head.

- Bring your awareness to your inner self. Place your hands in whatever position that is comfortable for you—resting easily at your side, behind you, or gently in front of you. Remain still but alert.

- As you begin walking, start with a slow pace, paying attention to the sensation of your feet and legs as they move. Feel the heaviness, lightness, tingling, pressure, or even pain if it's present. Notice your sensations rather than your breath or a mantra. Be present in your body right now.

- Be mindful of the sensations that happen in your knees as you lift your feet and place them back down on the floor or the earth. Sense each step fully as you walk in a relaxed, comfortable way to the end of your path.

- When you arrive at your chosen stopping point, pause for a moment. Feel your whole body standing, letting your senses be awake. Turn to face the other direction.

- Before you begin walking, pause again and notice the sensations of your body: the heaviness, lightness, tingling, pressure, or pain if there is any present. Notice how your body feels in this space and how your feet support the weight of your total body.

- You may find it helpful to close your eyes before you begin walking to sense even more deeply. If pain or emotions arise as you are present in this exercise, stand still and bring awareness, kindness, and presence to yourself as you notice these conditions and let them wash through you.

- As your mind wanders—planning, judging, or worrying—gently turn your attention to the next step or the next sensation. No matter how long your mind has wandered, it is always refreshed as you bring it back to the attention of self.

- As you continue your walking meditation, you may alter your pace to one that feels right for you at this time.

- As you complete this meditation, come to a stop. Notice the changes in your body, breath, and mind. Feel the sensations in all the parts of your body that have supported you throughout this walk or stance. Give thanks to yourself for this attention, and gratitude for the embodiment of your personal self-care.

As Thích Nhất Hạnh teaches, "The miracle is not to walk on water. It is to walk on this earth with awareness." By combining movement and awareness, walking meditations are a simple way to tap in to the MBC.

Guided Imagery to Create a Safe Place for Healing

Good for: chronic pain, releasing tension, stress relief

Guided imagery in meditation is a powerful way to access inner peace, relaxation, and healing. This exercise is best done twice daily, at regular times, so that you can create a safe place to retreat to, in order to calm yourself throughout the day. With repetition, you'll find it easier to use guided imagery in times of stress, pain, and discomfort.

Let's begin.

- Find a comfortable position, either lying or sitting down, with your head, neck, and spine supported and at ease. Feel free to adapt with pillows and bolsters to create a comfortable resting space.

- Gently close your eyes and notice the softening of your face and jaw, releasing the tension behind your eyes and allowing yourself to settle into a comfortable, supported position.

- Begin by taking a few slow, deep, easy breaths. Make no effort; allow the breathing to be as natural as possible.

- As you breathe in, allow this breath to move to any part of the body that is tight or sore.

- Release any tension as you exhale, breathing it out.

- If any emotions or thoughts come to mind, you can also release them as you exhale. Let your mind be calm.

- Now imagine a place where you feel calm and peaceful—a somewhere from your past or somewhere that you've never been but can imagine feels safe and peaceful.

- Allow this place to become real to you. In your mind's eye, look around and become familiar with the sounds, sights, and textures of anything you reach out to touch.

- Feel the surface that you're sitting or lying upon—the texture of the ground beneath you, whether it's sand, grass, or the soft pine needles that cover the forest floor.

- Notice any smells, whether they be a rich fragrance of peony, pine, or salty sea air.

- Feel the sunlight or gentle wind that may touch your skin, ruffling the hairs on your arms and legs. Perhaps you feel the mystic power of moonbeams that flow down on you.

- Take in the rich abundance with all your senses and become more attuned to your safe, special place. Feel gratitude for the beauty and the healing vibrance of it all.

- Let the beauty and the peace of this special place penetrate each and every cell, soaking into your skin, down to your muscles, nerves, tissue, and bones, and to the very center of your soul.

- Soak for as long as you need to in this stillness, beauty, and peace. Keep your eyes closed for as long as you wish, noticing how your body, mind, and breath feel.

- When you are ready, become aware of the sounds in the room and slowly blink your eyes awake and give thanks to yourself for taking this time for healing.

Know that you can come back to this place whenever you want to bring your body into alignment and find peace and comfort without pain. Simply find a quiet time and location, and return to this special place that you have created for healing.

Meditation
for Acceptance

Good for: chronic pain, releasing tension, stress relief

We can't control people, things, or experiences that come up as we go about our lives. But we can control how we respond. Each moment is an opportunity to accept, open, and expand—or to reject, retract, and shrink. Every time we practice acceptance, we open to who we are becoming in this world. And every time we withdraw from the moment, we close ourselves off to life and our souls. Choosing to fully accept each moment is both a daily practice and a lifelong journey.

Let's begin.

- Sit or lie in a comfortable position. You may want to close your eyes so you aren't distracted.

- Bring your attention to your breath, breathing in and breathing out.

- Become aware of any tension in your body. Breathe into that area for a moment and notice any thoughts that arise.

- See them like clouds in the sky, coming and going. You are the vast, blue, endless sky. Like the sky, you are unchanging as the clouds come and go.

- Let any thoughts that arise simply float up and out.

- If any emotions surface, feel and experience them—don't resist or fight.

- Emotions are not permanent. When we create room for feelings, they move through us. When fear, anxiety, or unrest arises, let yourself be with it.

- Accept your feelings and let them move through you, opening yourself up to the deep space and stillness within. You will then have room for love, light, and peace to come in.

- Breathing in and breathing out, just let it be.

- You are here, now, alive.

- Feel your heart beating.

- Feel your body expand as your breath comes in. Feel your body relax as the breath recedes.

- Breathing in and breathing out, accept this moment fully, as it is.

- Bring your awareness back to the present moment.

- Let your breathing deepen. Feel your body being supported as you breathe in and out.

- When you're ready, gently open your eyes.

You can use this acceptance meditation to soothe yourself anytime you feel unrest. Just take a few minutes to breathe, put your hands over your heart area, and let love, comfort, and ease fill your heart and soul.

Rev. Catherine Duncan, 2020.

Meet Your Pain
with Peace

Good for: chronic pain, headaches, joint pain,
nerve pain, releasing tension, stress relief

Being at peace with severe pain is difficult. Fortunately, pain can be reframed using mind-body techniques. This is a 20-minute guided meditation using imagery and relaxation. If at any time the images or words don't sit well within you, release them in a neutral way and substitute your own as you continue to deepen your sense of calm and quiet.

Let's begin.

- Find a quiet, relaxed space. Settle in to begin your journey inward to find a place of peace with pain.

- Gently close your eyes and take slow, comfortable breaths while noticing the sounds around you. Feel the sense of support from where you are sitting or lying down. Notice the breath move effortlessly into your nose and out through your mouth.

- Imagine that your pain is an incredible windstorm or hurricane of water, wind, and rain.

- Prepare to journey through the storm to a place that's like the eye of a hurricane—a place of calm where the winds are far away from your peaceful sanctuary.

- Gather any equipment, clothes, and supplies that you will need as you journey toward the center of the storm. You will be walking through it with only your intuition and internal compass to guide you. Let the fury of your pain drives you to this calm place in the center of the storm.

- Visualize a wooden door stands before you—it's solid and deeply carved. There is no handle or doorknob that you can see. You want to step through this door, but you don't know how it opens. Yet, somehow, you know that this door will open when you are ready.

- Wait, with a sense of calm and inner strength, knowing that the door will open. And suddenly, it does.

- You are immediately transported past the noisy, lightning-filled wall of the storm that pulls on your tissues and pounds in your ears as you push your way through it. You know how this storm feels—it is your pain. Move beyond it now!

- Suddenly, you are past the storm, and you know that you are safe. Your breathing is calm and relaxed—slow, deep, and regular.

- As you look at your surroundings, you notice a sense of familiarity. You've been here before. You wander around in amazement and wonder at this joyful, familiar place that wraps you with love and security.

- Feeling calm and protected, you find a comfortable place to sit and rest your body. You feel nestled and secure as you notice the beautiful colors, the wonderful smells, and the rich, resonant sounds that move beneath you and around you.

- As you rest, you hear the sound of the wind in the water and the crashing somewhere in the distance. It is far, far away from this secure, peaceful space of comfort.

- You are unafraid and breathing in a way that nourishes and nurtures you. Let the calm and peacefulness move throughout your entire body.

CONTINUED

- Feel yourself nodding off into a deep, comforting sleep, knowing that, somehow, as you are resting, you will find healing in this place beyond the storm.

- Notice that the storm is quieting and that there are fewer raindrops, less water swirling, and less wind blowing in the distance as you slumber even deeper.

- As you rest, you feel the sun shining its warmth and clearing the distant storm. That soothing warmth is massaging and easing your muscles and bones as you rest and heal.

- Allow yourself to slowly awaken in this healing place.

- As you prepare to leave your special place, feel secure in your knowledge that it lies within and can be accessed anytime you have your own personal storm. You know the secret of opening the door.

- Think about what you want to take with you—something that you found here that helps you feel calm and quiet, that gives you a sense of relief and rejuvenation.

- You know that when you journey back to this special place and open the door, you will find your peace and relief.

- Take a deep, comfortable breath and bring yourself back to the here and now. Gently blink your eyes awake, notice the sounds of the room and the sensation of the surface that supports you.

- Breathe in a sense of calm and relaxation.

Use this exercise whenever you feel the storm of your pain or emotions, knowing that you can easily come back to this place through the special door and experience relief, wonder, and calm.

Zoom-Out Meditation to Decrease Pain

Good for: headaches, chronic pain, joint pain, nerve pain

Sometimes when we are overwhelmed by our emotions, a wider perspective helps us become aware of what's in our control and what's not. It lets us simply accept what we cannot change. The zoom-out technique can shift us from being controlled by our emotions to being free to deal with our lives with compassion, care, and acceptance. When you zoom out, it can help you stop spiraling into negative thoughts and emotions and let you know that you are not alone in the world.

Let's begin.

- Find a comfortable place to sit or lie down, using pillows and bolsters to help your body to relax.

- Notice your breath as you begin to calm your nervous system.

- Gently bring up any negative thoughts, emotions, or feelings of pain that you are experiencing right now.

- Shift your attention from your breath to your right hand. Imagine that the thumb on your right hand is filled with space. You may choose to fill the space with any color that comes to mind.

- Now allow your perception to zoom out. Imagine the space filling your palms and the back of your hands, extending into your wrists, lower arms, elbows, upper arms, shoulders, underarms, waist, hips, thighs, knees, calf muscles, ankles, heels, the soles of your feet, the top of your feet, and all your toes.

- Imagine connecting all the space between your eyes, the back of your neck, the bridge of your nose, the back of your head, between your temples, and in your forehead and brain.

- Zoom out even more.

- Now connect the space inside your lungs, inside the bronchial tubes as you inhale and exhale, the space inside your throat, and your nose.

- Zoom out even further.

- Imagine that your body from the diaphragm down is filled with space. This includes your stomach, your belly, and your pelvis, down to your feet and toes.

- Let your whole body be filled with space, adding any color that comes to mind.

- Feel your entire body being filled with air when you inhale and filled with space when you exhale.

- Sense the space inside and around your whole body, above your head and beneath your chair or supported surface, in front of you and to your sides.

- Zoom out more.

- Let yourself be filled with all the sounds around you, including the sound of the voice of this recording, any sounds outside the room, and any sounds that your clothes make as they rustle against your skin.

- Now observe yourself as if you were above your body and looking down at yourself through the lens of the camera.

- Zoom out and see yourself and your surroundings. Zoom out more to see the space that surrounds your neighborhood and the region where you live, connecting you to those you love.

- See your loved ones as they smile at you. As you visualize these people who care for you, shift your attention to one person in particular, according to what you need most at this

CONTINUED

very moment. Perhaps it is safety, kindness, wisdom, or a gentle hug. Allow yourself to feel this person's unconditional love while they smile at you. They don't need to be alive, just present in your heart.

- Notice the feeling within your body, breath, and mind as you bring your attention back into the room you are in.

- Feel the love and support that you were able to zoom out and gather up and bring back to yourself.

- As you continue to use this zoom-out technique, you will be able to shift your attention faster and more completely and effortlessly.

- Now, repeating the zoom, imagine looking at yourself just as you are right now from above through the lens of the camera. Zoom out a little bit more to see yourself in the context of the room that you are in. Now take that camera even higher and imagine the building you are in, the neighborhood, the city, and the universe.

- Keep your images strong. Allow yourself to smell, touch, and feel each sensation, environment, and person that you zoom out to meet.

- Bring your attention back to your breath. Notice the sounds of the room, the sensations of your body, the calm of your mind, and the peace of your breath.

Practice this exercise anytime you feel that you need to step back and see things from a wider perspective, letting it help make your negative emotions feel more manageable.

Kindness Meditation

Good for: chronic pain, releasing tension, stress relief

I love this quote by poet Stephen Levine: "Letting go of our suffering is the hardest work we will ever do. It is also the most fruitful. To heal means to meet ourselves in a new way—in the newness of each moment where all is possible and nothing is limited to the old." By learning to cultivate kindness, forgiveness, and compassion toward ourselves, we can start to heal our pain. This kindness meditation can help you do just that.

Let's begin.

- Sit or lie with the intention that for the next half hour, you will be enjoying and cultivating kindness and love toward yourself and others. Allow the events of the day to be released from your mind and body. Just let go of them and focus on your breath and your senses in the here and now.

- Take a few deep breaths to calm down your mind. Breathe in and be aware that you're breathing in. Breathe out and be aware that you're breathing out.

- After a few breaths, you may find that your mind is wandering. This is natural, so don't resist it or show any resentment. Observe the thoughts that come and go.

- Bring your attention back to your breath and anchor the breathing in and breathing out, calmly and peacefully.

- Visualize your awareness as a ball of golden light. Allow it to sweep around your head, ears, eyes, and jaw, releasing any tension or tightness that is found in these areas.

- Gently shift your awareness to your shoulders and neck, allowing them to relax and soften with the golden light, warming and releasing.

CONTINUED

- Allow this golden light to move across your shoulder joints down your arm, hands, and fingers.

- Bring your attention to your chest area. Let that golden light touch your heart, lungs, liver, pancreas, spleen, large and small intestines, abdomen, reproductive organs, and kidneys, to create vitality, and comfort.

- Spread this golden light of loving-kindness around your spinal cord, pelvis, thighs, legs, knees, feet, and toes, wrapping them with warmth, comfort, and love.

- Observe the feeling of softness and relaxation in all the muscles of your body, letting go of all the physical stresses within the skin, muscles, organs, and ligaments.

- Gently bring your awareness back to rest on the relaxation and the rhythm of the inhalation and exhalation as you observe the stillness within you.

- Allow your attention to move throughout your whole physical, mental, and emotional system, seeking out peace, forgiveness, and love.

- Allow that golden light of grace to move through the feeling of forgiveness and compassion as you breathe in and breathe out gently, calmly, and with love.

- As you bask in this golden light of grace, mentally say to yourself, "May my heart be peaceful and free from negative emotions." Repeat it slowly a few times and notice any feelings that come from the center of your heart.

- Continue feeling this golden light of grace as you mentally say, "May my mind be happy." Think of your mind as being relaxed and happy, and repeat this phrase to yourself until you feel as though it is rooted deeply within your consciousness.

- Be aware of the strength and sensation in your physical body, and bring your attention to your solar plexus area. Mentally say, "May my body be healthy and strong. May I be well and happy."

- As you mentally repeat these phrases, let this energy move through your mind, and feel your anger, hatred, jealousy, frustration, and anxiety releasing and transmuting into golden light.

- Take a few comfortable, easy breaths and allow your golden grace of loving-kindness to include those close to you who are in need of love, care, and protection. Bring to mind these people you love and see them happy, radiant, healthy, and peaceful.

- Keeping your awareness of calm and peaceful feelings, send this compassion and loving-kindness to someone who is difficult and problematic to you at work or elsewhere. Consider that this person wants to be happy and peaceful just like you.

- Mentally say, "May your heart be peaceful and free from negative emotions. May your mind be happy. May your body be healthy and strong. May you be well and happy."

CONTINUED

- Spread this loving-kindness to include your neighbors and those you don't know. Mentally say to all those known and unknown, "May your heart be peaceful and free from negative emotions. May your mind be happy. May your body be healthy and strong. May you be well and happy."

- Take a few deep, easy breaths, and give yourself thanks and appreciation for taking the time to nourish, heal, and calm your nervous system.

- Begin to notice the sensation of the surface that supports you, the sounds that are around you, and your body feeling peaceful and at rest.

- Take a final comfortable and easy breath, slowly blinking your eyes awake and coming back to your room refreshed and at peace.

Remember that treating yourself with kindness and compassion is one of the first steps toward healing.

Deepening Awareness

*Good for: chronic pain, headaches, nerve pain,
releasing tension, stress relief*

This meditation allows you the opportunity to move deeper into the sensation and quality of your physical body. You'll be using imagery and inner sensing to pay attention to the quality of your breath as it moves throughout your body.

Let's begin.

- Sit or lie down in a comfortable position and bring your attention to your breath. Take three deep breaths, allowing the inhale to fill your body completely and letting your body relax on the surface that supports you as you exhale.

- Bring your attention to your body, and imagine breathing into your feet and becoming aware of any sensations or lack of sensations there.

- Imagine the bones and muscles beneath the skin. Move your attention and breathe into your lower legs, first one and then the other.

- Be aware of the bones running between your ankle and your knees, of the calf muscles in the skin of the lower legs. Notice any sensations in this area—if you are feeling any discomfort, try to notice it without judgment.

- Let your breath fill one leg and then the other. From there, breathe into your upper legs, moving from the knees into the thighs and then the hips. Become aware of how your legs are attached to the pelvis.

- Imagine that you can feel the blood flow from your feet, moving all the way up both of your legs, including through the bones that support the nerves, vessels, and muscles.

CONTINUED

- Bring your breath into your hips and pelvis area. If you feel any areas of discomfort, breathe more deeply into those areas. Notice that the pelvis is a bowl that supports your spine as it rises up from the center.

- Continue taking easy, slow breaths, breathing once again from your feet, up the legs, into the pelvis, and around the base of the spine.

- Notice any areas where your breath might have been less smooth, or caught up on a bubble of discomfort. Notice without out a story attached to the sensation.

- Breathe into your lower back and into the deep layers of the muscles attached to the bones of the hip. Notice if the breath is smooth or tight as you breathe through the thickness of the back muscles.

- Let your breath move up and around the spine, the rib cage, and into the shoulders—including the shoulder blades that support your arms.

- Breathe through each fingertip and imagine the breath moving through the hands, up the forearms, into the biceps, and swirling into the shoulders.

- Notice how the breath feels different from the fingertips to the shoulder blades.

- Notice if the breath feels lighter or denser in any part of the arms.

- Now bring your attention to your neck and head.

- Observe any sensations that arise as you are breathing through dense muscle tissue and the vessels that nourish your entire system. As you breathe, fill your lungs and let your chest open and expand beyond its physical barriers. Become aware of the connection between your lower and upper body.

- Breathe in through your lips and allow that breath to fill your throat, jaw, and face.

- Notice how the breath moves through your face as compared to the shoulders and lower back. If you have any areas of discomfort in your neck, jaw, or face, bring your breath there and notice and release it.

- Breathe into your head, being aware of the sides of your temples, your ears, the bones of your skull, and your scalp.

- Notice any sensations around your lips, tongue, and teeth. Breathe into the areas around your eyes and behind your eyes. Notice how the breath relaxes the eyes, as well as the face muscles, jaw, and tongue.

- Feel the life-force energy that runs through your blood, your nerve endings, and every cell and molecule within your entire system.

- Breathe into your whole body and become aware of any physical sensations and emotions that arise as you bring awareness to each part of your physical system.

CONTINUED

- And finally, move your breath from your toes, up through the entire body, and out the top of the head.

- Feel the sensation of gratitude and stillness that this breath has brought you. Allow yourself to notice the sounds around you and the sensation of the surface that supports you as you slowly blink your eyes awake and come back to the room, refreshed and alert.

The deeper the awareness you have of your body, the easier it will be to understand—and manage—your pain. Use this exercise whenever you need to get in touch with the physical sensations of your whole body.

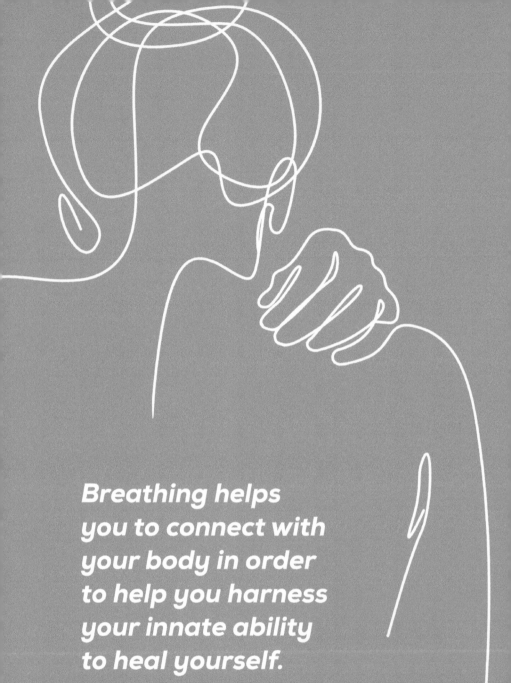

Breathing helps you to connect with your body in order to help you harness your innate ability to heal yourself.

CHAPTER FIVE

Remember to Breathe

Breath is essential to life. It's one of the first things you did when you were born, and it's one of the last things you'll do before you pass. In this chapter, you will explore a variety of techniques designed to decrease stress and minimize pain. Learning to breathe with conscious awareness can be a valuable tool in helping you restore balance to your mind and body.

Meet Richie

Richie, a 32-year-old patient, was referred from a neurologist who knew I specialized in patients with complex pain. As a result of a brain-stem injury when Richie was three months old, his cognitive skills were those of an eight-year-old, and he was suffering from severe migraine headaches four to five times a week. But when I met with Richie and his mom, I discovered that his migraine headaches actually went away when he read the Bible. He was devoutly religious, felt very connected to God, and believed that this was a time in which God relieved his headaches. I was excited that he had found a way to get rid of his migraines. The problem was that as soon as he stopped reading the Bible, the migraine came back. Though he couldn't spend the whole day reading, he had tapped into something that helped him overcome the physiological effects of a migraine headache. Anyone who has had migraines knows that this type of headache is hard to treat.

I decided to use a technique that would eventually get Richie comfortable with using his breath to help relieve his migraines: a process of biofeedback called heart rate variability (HRV). This technique measures your autonomic nervous system and teaches you how to control both the sympathetic and parasympathetic activities. I look at it as a balancing type of exercise that is controlled by the breath.

My favorite way to use HRV is HeartMath, a type of biofeedback to help people reframe their breathing. It's based on research that shows how feelings of love, care, appreciation, or pride can trigger cells in the brain to produce neurochemicals such as serotonin and dopamine. Using this specific technique allowed me to make the connection between reading the Bible and heart breathing, because that's how Richie created pain relief for himself.

I used a visual biofeedback system that showed a green light when Richie's breath was balanced and coherent. When his breath was out of sync, the light turned red. Richie would place his hand on his heart and read the Bible while breathing in for six counts and out for six counts, and watching that the monitor stayed green. He was able to notice that his shoulders became relaxed, his breath was calmer, and his headaches began to leave.

Eventually Richie was able to perform heart breathing as soon as he felt his migraines begin. Richie still loves to read the Bible for his personal joy, but he is able to reduce and eliminate his migraines just by using heart breathing techniques. He was able to reframe the situation around his migraine and understand that he had control over his body by breathing in a way that balanced his nervous system.

I was so impressed that he had figured out his own way to stop his migraines in their tracks with his reading. My job was to help him understand that he already had full control over his pain. By using biofeedback and external devices, he was able to see what he was doing and sustain that feeling of relaxation and joy. When I followed up with his mom several months later, she said he was able to move out to a group home because his migraines were under control and he had less fear about living away from her.

Breathwork

In all the years of working with the chronic pain population, I have found breathwork to be the most potent and sustainable exercise for reducing pain and calming the nervous system. The way you breathe sends signals to your brain, which can either ramp up or calm down your limbic system.

If you have persistent pain, it's common to try to distance yourself from your body. It hurts, and you want out. Breathing helps you connect with your body, in order to help you harness your innate ability to heal yourself. By consciously working with your breath and becoming aware of how you breathe, you can influence the parasympathetic nervous system and change your HRV. This alters brain wave activities, and changes the chemical structure and even the neural structure of your brain.

When you have pain and stress, your breathing tends to be shallow. It's a response that many people are unaware of—small sips of air throughout the day. When you take small breaths, you are overusing your neck and shoulder muscles in order to get enough oxygen to survive. The conundrum is that this unconscious, shallow, upper-chest breathing creates a stress response.

Dr. Herbert Benson at Harvard Medical School developed a relaxation response to reduce shallow breathing due to pain or stress. The foundation of this technique is deep, slow breathing. A 2012 study on breathing and pain perception, published in *Pain Medicine*, found that this type of breathing reduced negative feelings, including tension, anger, and depression, as well as pain. Both acute pain and chronic pain can be treated with a variety of breathing techniques.

The Key to Survival

Breathing is part of a larger chain reaction within your body that helps you to integrate all of your systems. As you can imagine, without breath, there is no life. Your brain is very interested in living, so it will dismiss anything in your body that keeps it from sustaining life. That means if you're breathing in a shallow way that doesn't provide enough oxygen to your brain, the brain might shut down some of the organs that are taking some of the oxygen. That might mean more tension in your muscles, or that some of the vessels that bring blood flow to your organs will also get squeezed so that the brain can get enough oxygen. This squeezing can be incredibly painful, especially in the nerves.

When you take a breath in your lungs, this is called inspiration. The diaphragm drops down, making the chest cavity a little bigger, as your muscles pull your ribs up and out of the way, letting air fill up the all the microscopic air sacs called alveoli. In the lungs, this oxygen hops onto your red blood cells to be delivered to the capillaries, veins, and heart, and then moves into the systemic arteries that deliver it throughout your body. Breathing is unique because it's both conscious and unconscious. The ability to control breath is located in the brain and is affected by emotions, thoughts, and even the structure of the body. You can use mindfulness to manage your pain. How often have you heard somebody tell you to take a big, deep breath when you have pain? Did it help? The science says that it probably did.

Best Through the Nose

Ancient yogis and researchers all agree that breathing through the nose has tremendous benefits for the body. This is one function of the body that you can consciously choose to control. The nose filters the air that we breathe, making sure particles are trapped in the cilia that line the nostrils, and safely allowing the moistened, temperature-controlled air to enter the lungs. When the filtered air enters your lungs, oxygen is pumped into your bloodstream and circulated through all of your organs and vessels. Then the oxygen gets exchanged for carbon dioxide, which is a waste material from the body, and this is what you exhale.

When poor breathing has become a habit, the muscles that lift your ribs and expand your lungs become weak, causing your lung capacity to shrink. Breathing through your nose allows you to take deeper breaths into the lower lungs. This allows the oxygen to stay in the lungs longer, which means that more carbon dioxide can be exchanged, thereby helping rid your body of cellular waste.

Another benefit of bringing breath into the lower lungs is that your parasympathetic, or calming, nerve receptors are there. They send a chemical message to your brain that helps you become less stressed and more relaxed. The short, upper-chest breathing that's common with mouth breathers can activate the sympathetic nerve receptors in the upper chest, which cause the fight-or-flight reaction in your body.

Breathing through the nose forces you to slow down your breath. Your sinuses produce nitric oxide, which protects you against bacteria and viruses, boosts the immune system, stabilizes your blood pressure, and has a cardiovascular protective effect. It also improves sleep, memory, focus, and concentration. Like any new habit, nasal breathing may be challenging when you first begin, so take it slowly, trust the process, and notice the benefits.

Breathing Exercises

Changing the way you breath can be challenging. I recommend that you record the breathing exercises so you can relax and pay attention to how you breathe. You may find that some of these techniques seem difficult to master. Start slowly, giving yourself plenty of time to adapt to this new way of using your body and breath. Once you have done each exercise a few times, you may find that you can easily remember the instructions.

Basic Breath Awareness

Good for: chronic pain, joint pain, releasing tension, stress relief

If you watch pets or babies breathe, you'll notice that they are breathing properly—with their tummies rising on the in breath and falling on the out breath. If you're not used to breathing through your diaphragm, this exercise will guide you through basic breathwork that will allow you to breathe as nature intended.

Let's begin.

- The easiest way to start learning how to breathe properly is by lying down on your back. You can have your legs out straight, or bent with a pillow underneath your knees for comfort.

- Let your arms fall to your sides naturally and feel your shoulder blades in contact with the surface you are lying on.

- Put one hand on your abdomen just below the rib cage and the other hand on your chest.

- Inhale slowly. Focus on your abdomen coming up and pressing into your hand. The other hand, on your chest, should stay still.

- If you have a long-term habit of breathing out of sync, it may help you to place a pillow or a book underneath the hand on your abdomen. This allows you to feel your breath more deeply as you inhale.

- Exhale smoothly while tightening your abdominal muscles. You'll feel the pressure under the hand over your abdominal area decrease.

Practice this morning and evening for a few days so that you get accustomed to the way it feels. You'll then be more likely to notice when you're not breathing naturally throughout the day.

Belly Breathing

Good for: chronic pain, headaches, joint pain,
nerve pain, releasing tension, stress relief

Diaphragmatic breathing is often called belly breathing. This is a gentle and easy breathing exercise that allows you to get in touch with how breath can easily move in and out of your body. This is one of the most beneficial breathing techniques for chronic pain. It helps with relaxation, distraction, and calming anxiety and stress.

If you have been an upper chest breather most of your life, diaphragmatic breathing may feel somewhat stressful. As with the previous exercise, it helps to place a book or a magazine on top of your belly in order to have something physical to push against as you breathe into your diaphragm.

Let's begin.

- Find a comfortable place to lie down or sit, where you are well supported. If lying down, you may find it easier to place a pillow beneath your knees, or even place your legs on an ottoman at a 90-degree angle with a pillow under your head. If you're sitting, allow your knees to be bent, with your shoulders, neck, and head relaxed.

- Place one hand on the upper chest and the other below the rib cage.

- Breathe in slowly through your nose, allowing your stomach to move out against your hand. Try to keep the hand on your chest as still as possible.

- As you exhale through pursed lips—like you're trying to blow out a candle—tighten the stomach muscles while the air moves up from your belly and out of the mouth.

- Continue breathing for 5 to 10 minutes, allowing the breath to flow in and out beneath your lower hand.

- Allow yourself some time to become comfortable with this technique, especially if this type of breathing is new to you.

I often call this technique rescue breathing. You can do it for 5 to 10 minutes three to four times a day, whenever you're in pain.

Rib Cage Breathing

Good for: chronic pain, headaches, joint pain, nerve pain, releasing tension, stress relief

In order to take a full breath, the rib cage has to expand with the help of the intercostal muscles (the muscles in between each rib) to allow the lungs to fully expand. This expansion takes place front to back and side to side. Think of the rib cage area as a collapsible wire basket. The in breath expands the wire mesh out, and the exhalation allows the mesh to collapse on itself.

As we age—and with pain and some diseases—the muscles between the ribs get weaker, so the rib cage doesn't expand to its normal breath and width. This exercise will help strengthen the muscles for breathing while allowing you to tune in to the patterns of your breath and learn how to train your body to give yourself the best breath possible.

For this exercise, you'll need an elastic therapy band or belt that fits around your back and chest. It's important to feel what you're doing in order to understand how the breath moves through your body. It's easiest to sit tall as you do this exercise, but if pain makes that difficult, you can do it lying down on a bed, a couch, or the floor.

Let's begin.

- Become comfortable on a chair or lying down. Wrap either an elastic band or belt around your torso and then place your hands at the sides of the rib cage, just above the floating ribs.

- Relax your back so that it's slightly rounded, with your shoulders forward, in order to keep you from chest breathing.

- Take a deep breath and hold it.

- While you are holding your breath, draw in your abdominal muscles. This creates pressure in the inflated lungs, and pushes the ribs outward and into your hands so that you can feel them.

- Maintain that pressure as long as the breath can be comfortably held. Notice if your shoulders are trying to get into the action, and if they are, let them relax and be at ease.

- Slowly release your breath, with your hands pushing inward on the ribs to feel the rib cage close.

- Notice how that felt while breathing in and out. Repeat this two to five times.

Sometimes this type of breathing can cause a feeling of light-headedness or hyperventilation. Make sure that you don't hold your breath too long, and stop if it feels uncomfortable.

Alternate Nostril Breathing

Good for: chronic pain, releasing tension, stress relief

Alternate nostril breathing is said to balance both the right and left brain hemispheres, and the nervous and hormonal systems. It very quickly brings the mind into Theta—the thrifty, dreamy brain state that happens just before sleep. This method can be done quite quickly to calm your system and reduce your feelings of stress and anxiety, while at the same time increasing your energy.

Let's begin.

- Sit with your back straight and gently close your lips. If you are wearing glasses, remove them.

- Find a position that allows you to support your right arm as you gently place your index and middle finger together on your forehead, between your eyebrows. You may find it comfortable to support your right elbow with your left forearm.

- Start by closing your left nostril with your little or index finger. Inhale through your right nostril to the count of four. Pause for the count of four and exhale for the count of four.

- Repeat this five times to practice how this breath feels in your body.

- Release your left nostril and close your right nostril with your right thumb. Inhale to the count of four and exhale to the count of four, completing the cycle five times. Don't force your breath—if you need to take a break, breathe through both nostrils and then continue when you are ready.

- Now close your right nostril with your right thumb and inhale through your left nostril. Then close your left nostril with your ring or little finger, and lift your thumb to exhale through your right nostril. Then inhale through the same nostril. Close your right nostril with your thumb and lift your finger to exhale through your left nostril. Try to keep your inhalation and exhalation to the count of four.

- If this process causes you any distress, inhale and exhale naturally.

- This is one round. You'll do three to five rounds. You can build up the number of rounds as you practice this exercise and become more confident.

- When you have repeated five rounds, rest your hands on your thighs with your palms facing upward. Take natural and normal breaths through both nostrils and be mindful of any changes in your energy, thoughts, and emotions.

I recommend starting slowly with short sessions and building up over time. If at any time you find that your stress level is increasing while doing this breathing technique, stop and breathe normally. You can also switch the hand that is holding the nostrils open and closed.

Calming Breath

Good for: chronic pain, releasing tension, stress relief

This exercise, also known as 4-7-8 breath, is designed to increase your energy while at the same time decreasing pain and fatigue. It can also be used whenever you have any type of internal tension, especially in a situation where you are ready to react rather than respond. It's quickly mastered and easily done. When doing this breath work, I recommend setting a timer every hour or two, throughout the day.

Research has shown that this simple, pain-relief breathwork is useful in managing stress. It calms the nervous system and can be used when anything upsetting happens or when you're trying to fall asleep.

Let's begin.

• Place the tip of your tongue against the upper front teeth and keep it there for the entire exercise. Don't push hard; just gently rest the tongue.

• Exhale completely through your mouth, making a sound like "whoosh" or "haaaah."

• Close your mouth and inhale quietly through your nose to a mental count of four.

• Hold your breath for the count of seven.

• Exhale completely through your mouth, making the same sound as before, to the count of eight.

• This is one breath. Now inhale again and repeat the cycle three more times, for a total of four breaths.

I recommend that you only do four breaths at a time for the first month of practice. If you feel a little light-headed when you first breathe this way, don't be concerned—it's a new skill, and the feeling will pass.

The 4-7-8 ratio is important because it's a natural tranquilizer for the nervous system.

Resilient Attitude Breathing

Good for: chronic pain, releasing tension, stress relief

Chronic pain can affect attitudes about yourself and the world around you. The quality of your thoughts and emotions determines the instructions that your heart sends to your brain. In order to change your relationship to your thoughts, feelings, and body, you must practice shifting your attitudes and beliefs in a sustainable and consistent way.

In this breathing exercise you will be reframing your thoughts and emotions. With practice, you will begin to rewire the intricate network of your miles of living nerves. By learning how to restructure the attitudes that may be unhelpful in your journey toward resilience, you will have a greater control over your body and mind.

Let's begin.

- The first step is to recognize attitudes or feelings that you're ready to change. It's essential to have a feeling of readiness in order for this to succeed. These attitudes could be anxiety, sadness, despair, depression, self-judgment, guilt, anger, or feeling overwhelmed. Anything that feels distressing and disturbing to you is fair game for change.

- Once you've identified a particular attitude that you want to change, you'll need to find a replacement attitude. For example, if the attitude/feeling that you are ready to change is anxiety, you'll be breathing a feeling or statement of calm and balance. The breath is slow and purposeful through the heart, with kindness and care.

- Breathe out the negative attitude and breathe in the replacement attitude. It may take 10 to 15 times breathing this attitude in and out through your heart for you to feel a difference.

CONTINUED

- As you breathe your replacement attitude, it's important to take the drama out of the attitude. Allow the attitude to be neutral, rather than fired up and filled with history and negativity.

- Breathe in the new attitude through your heart until you feel something shift within you.

- Continue to practice this attitude, breathing to address feelings and thoughts that are out of sync with your feelings of resilience, calm, and peace.

- Learn to recognize the moment when the sensation and attachment to the attitude/feeling that you are replacing shifts into something that is either neutral or positive.

- As new attitudes and feelings arise in your life, appreciate that your commitment to releasing and replacing will create new neural pathways with positive benefits.

REPLACEMENT ATTITUDES

As you move through this exercise, you may experience unwanted feelings. Below are some techniques to help you work through those emotions.

Stress: Breathe in a feeling of neutrality, letting go, chilling out.

Anxiety: Breathe in calm and balance.

Overwhelmed: Breathe in and mentally say, "I am safe, I am healing, everything is going to be okay."

Depression: Breathe in calm and peace.

Guilt: Breathe in compassion and nonjudgment.

Feeling the victim: Breathe in gratitude and surrender.

Focused Heart Breathing

Good for: chronic pain, headaches, nerve pain, stress relief

This exercise will teach you how to access the power of positive emotions through a heart-centered breathing approach. It's important to practice this exercise on a regular basis in order to retrain your brain toward happiness, peace, and joy. Negative thoughts are automatic, but positive thoughts have to be learned and installed in order to become unconscious.

Before you do the following exercise, think of a memory or recall a place that brings you joy, happiness, pride, or peace. These are the emotions that allow for chemical changes in the brain that are activated by your breath and create shifts within your physical, mental, and emotional system. When you are stressed or in pain, these thoughts aren't easily accessed, so it's important to practice them ahead of time so you can access them on the fly. If you can't think of something pleasant, a neutral phrase such as "inner peace" or "I am safe" works just as well.

Let's begin.

- Find a comfortable and relaxed position.

- Set a timer for five minutes.

- Place your hand over your heart, or just shift your focus to the area of your heart.

- Begin to breathe a little more slowly than usual, and imagine that the breath is coming in and out of your heart.

- Remember the positive emotion, feeling, or place that you have prepared for. Embrace that feeling to the best of your ability as you begin to breathe in and out of your heart.

- Continue focusing on this positive feeling as you continue to breathe for five minutes.

- When your mind wanders, bring your focus back to the breath that is moving in and out of your heart, activating your positive feelings of joy, care, or appreciation.

- As you continue to breathe, allow the feeling of care or appreciation to heal, nourish, and calm your own body.

- Radiate that same positive feeling of care to someone you love.

- Now radiate that feeling to anyone in the world who is in need of care, comfort, and love.

- Once you have performed your heart-breathing exercise, notice the changes and sensations throughout your body, mind, and breath.

Your mind will wander during this exercise, but just bring your attention back to the positive feeling in the awareness of your breath. At the end of five minutes, you will begin to radiate that same feeling of care and appreciation to those you love and those who are in need of care—even if you don't know who that is. Research has shown that radiating love and self-care through your system activates beneficial hormones and boosts your immune system.

Awareness of Breath
for Pain Relief

Good for: chronic pain, headaches, joint pain,
nerve pain, releasing tension, stress relief

Each moment, your breath is nourishing millions of cells in your body. By focusing consciously on your breath, you can access and empower the mind-body connection for pain relief, relaxation, and well-being. Using diaphragmatic breathwork, this exercise cultivates awareness through mindfulness for pain relief.

Let's begin.

- Find a comfortable place to sit or lie down.

- It may be helpful to place one hand on your upper chest and one hand on your belly.

- The correct breathing pattern is to fill the belly first, so that your hand on the belly feels that air filling your body before arriving in your upper chest. If this feels unnatural, just allow yourself to count your breaths and become more aware of how your body feels as you are nourishing it with oxygen.

- Begin by taking a deep belly breath in through your nose to the count of four.

- Now slowly breathe out to the count of eight, pursing your lips as though you are blowing out a candle.

- Repeat this again, paying attention to how the air feels at the back of your throat, in your nostrils, and on your lips as you inhale and exhale.

- Send your affection and care to this breath as it flows into your lungs, nourishing you with life force. Imagine that you are infusing this breath with kindness and love as you observe the inhalation and the exhalation.

- Have you noticed any changes to your breathing now that you've been paying attention to it? Is your breathing deep or shallow? Are you breathing slowly, rapidly, gently, or sharply? Observe your breathing pattern without changing it, just becoming aware of the peace, warmth, and healing that your breath is bringing to your whole self.

- Continue noticing your breath as it moves in and out of your whole body.

- Inhale your breath to any parts of your body that feel a sense of discomfort or disease.

- As you exhale your breath from this place of discomfort, imagine that you are releasing any feelings that impact your sense of well-being.

- Continue to inhale and exhale on any parts of your body that you sense need extra care and compassion. Take as long as you need.

- Pause for 30 seconds or longer as your body takes care of any areas of pain, discomfort, or disease.

- If your mind wanders, allow your breath to bring you back to your sense of purpose—healing, calming, and releasing.

- Let your breath align with your thoughts of healing, and feel how your mind and your breath can combine for releasing pain and discomfort.

- Take a purposeful breath and bring in healing, peace, and a color that feels right to you.

- Infuse all of your cells, muscles, bones, and blood with this healing color. If no color comes to mind, that's okay. There are no rules—just breath and intentional thought.

CONTINUED

- As you continue to breathe in and out, feel gratitude for the breath of life and the ability to listen to these words as you set an intention for healing and peace.

- Inhale peace and comfort to the count of four.

- Exhale through your mouth any thoughts, emotions, and negativity that may linger within your body to the count of eight.

- Continue to breathe normally again, noticing how naturally your body takes in and releases breath without thought.

- Now bring your awareness back to the room, if you feel ready. Notice the changes in your muscles, thoughts, emotions, and breath.

Spend a few moments allowing yourself to reflect on what thoughts and emotions came up as you did this meditation. Do you now feel a deeper awareness of how your pain manifests throughout your body?

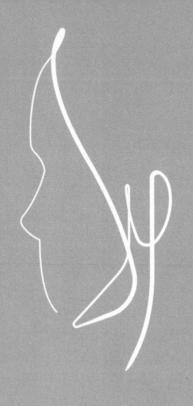

Restorative yoga can be transformative for people who suffer from persistent pain because it allows the body to be fully supported while the breath helps guide them into a deeper state of relaxation.

CHAPTER SIX

Make a Move

Movement is a key component in reducing pain. As I've mentioned motion is lotion, to keep your joints flexible and as healthy as can be. When you are experiencing persistent pain, fear is often a limiting factor in your ability to move. This chapter will show you restorative yoga movements that are safe, restorative, and designed to reduce stress and anxiety and support the body in healing.

Meet Joanie

Joanie was a tall, stunning woman with an incredible sense of humor. When I asked her about her relationship to her body, she replied, "Oh, we had a contentious divorce. I don't even have visiting rights."

It's easy to see why Joanie had these feelings toward her body. She had a connective tissue disorder called Ehlers-Danlos, which, for her, manifested as joint pain. Her ribs, wrists, and other joints slipped out of alignment on a regular basis, and she'd had 15 surgeries by the time I saw her. She rated her normal, everyday pain at 6 on a scale of 10. She often walled off the pain and pretended it really didn't exist. Anxiety, depression, and poor sleep are comorbidities of the disorder, and so she needed to learn tools to deal with those aspects of her disease as well.

Joanie's disconnected feelings toward her body were similar to those of my persistent pain clients. In her mind, her body had failed her and no longer deserved any respect or consideration. This disconnected relationship is quite common with chronic pain and is one of the most important things to heal in order to begin the process of recovery.

Lying on the table was uncomfortable for her lower back and neck, so I knew right away that restorative yoga would be one of the primary tools we would use in our therapy. Since it utilizes mindfulness, movement, reframing, and breathwork, yoga checks all the boxes. And, most importantly, Joanie was willing to give it a try.

I started with the concept that healing isn't always about being out of pain. Physical impairments and the constant chatter coming from her joints and muscles were her normal way of living. In order to get back into her body or become embodied, Joanie needed to restore the sacred connection between her body, mind, and spirit.

Her treatment started off very slowly. I began by simply supporting her ribs and neck with pillows and lifting her legs up onto a big therapy ball. I then opened her chest by placing a foam roller underneath her spine. I also supported her at the sides, adjusting with extra towels and extra lift to reduce any of the nerve pain coming from her neck. Bit by bit, we adapted and adjusted until her body was at complete rest.

From there she began to work with diaphragmatic breathing and affirmations. By doing breathwork and mindfully noticing her body using affirmations, she was able to find places on her body that had resisted change and movement because of fear and anger. Joanie was upfront that she didn't want to meditate, but she was fully committed to breathing with intention. She knew the two practices were very similar, but for some reason the only way she was going to do her exercises was to call them a different name. That worked for me.

Almost every time she tuned into her body with compassion and love, tears flowed. She told me that this type of exercise was like a mental balm. It eased her anxiety, decreased her pain, and allowed her to find new ways to move without fear of increasing her pain. The more time she spent breathing and resting in these restorative poses, the greater her forgiveness and compassion became. She realized that grief was a large part of her pain experience, and that learning how to grieve was a new skill.

With plenty of tissues, laughter, and creativity, Joanie was able to begin doing her own self-massage and daily exercise to increase her endurance and joint stabilization. She learned how to recognize fatigue and understood that rest is medicine. Joanie continues to have ongoing episodes, pain, and periodic surgeries, but the biggest change is her attitude toward her body and her pain. She told me that she's breathing, laughing, and resting her way through life.

Restorative Yoga

Restorative yoga is the ultimate mind-body connection practice. It involves movement and thought all rolled into one. As I mentioned before, yoga comes from a Sanskrit word that means "to yoke," dissolving the separation of body, mind, and spirit by integrating with the breath. Restorative yoga can be transformative for people who suffer from persistent pain, because it allows the body to be fully supported while the breath helps guide them into a deeper state of relaxation.

Restorative yoga is different from other yoga practices, which often create a competitive striving to work on your poses. In the supported poses, you use your breath to release tension and stress, and become aware of the places where you grip and hold on to that stress. While in the supported position, you can start to change the language about your pain and to soften the constant chatter of your nervous system.

Many people who have chronic pain experience disc, nerve, and degenerative conditions. One of the benefits of this type of yoga is that it teaches you how to relax your nervous system while promoting your own natural state of healing and repair. These supported poses are all very adaptable, but it's important to make sure that you've touched base with your health care practitioner first. And if you want to experience restorative yoga in a class, make sure that your teacher is certified in restorative techniques and is aware of your medical conditions.

Research from the NIH, Harvard, and the Cleveland Clinic has shown that yoga has been beneficial for improving quality of life for people experiencing cancer, asthma and breathing problems, and lower back pain. Interestingly, yoga has also recently been shown to be extremely beneficial for carpal tunnel syndrome.

Gentle Poses

In restorative yoga, props such as bolsters, blankets, pillows, towels, and belts are used to support the body in positions to provide longer stretches without any effort. Most of these positions are without gravity and should not be painful.

The idea behind using props is that it allows you to work at your own comfort level. They support your body without fear of strain and pain, allowing your mind to let go of its need to protect. Because of that, it becomes much easier to relax your thoughts and calm your body. Most poses start with three to five minutes, but the key is to be able to trust your body as you release your mind and your muscles.

It's so important that you don't push through pain—please take this out of your vocabulary.

You can buy specific yoga props, but can also use everyday household items. Foam rollers, towels, blankets, balls, long belts, and walls are all good props. Creativity will be your friend as you begin to understand the premise behind supporting, relaxing, and easing your body and mind.

Easy Resistance

If you're familiar with yoga, you may imagine that poses are all about getting wrapped up like a pretzel and finding yourself drenched in sweat with trembling limbs. Restorative yoga uses very different poses, done with easy resistance and in a pain-free manner. The goal is to create balance in the body, including organs, circulation, blood, breathing, and your energy system.

Never try to push into pain. The "no pain, no gain" theory is outdated and not useful now that we know more about pain neuroscience, and how the brain is alert to how we use our words and respond to pain in our system. Using phrases such as "bumping into your pain" or "nudging into the pain" while doing yoga poses allows the system to calm down.

These restorative poses promote more efficient breathing and also gently stretch and release the abdominal, intercostal, and paraspinal muscles, reducing tension throughout the body.

Yoga Poses

Movement, breath, and calming thoughts are all equally important in this practice. I encourage you to record yourself so you can practice these poses at your leisure.

Basic Rest Pose

Good for: chronic pain, releasing tension, stress relief

This basic rest pose is a simple restorative pose that is one of the first exercises I give to patients who are experiencing chronic pain. This is especially great to use when the lower back starts to get tight and there is excess tension or tightness in the psoas muscle, which is the muscle that gets tight when you sit for a long period of time.

Props: A long, folded blanket or beach towel for back support, one strap or long belt, one small ball or foam block for leg support, and one large dish towel or hand towel for neck and head support

Let's begin.

- On the floor, place a folded blanket the long way along the center of your mat.

- Lie down on it with the edge of the blanket filling in the curve of your lower back. If needed, place an additional hand or dish towel underneath your lower back to start. Place the towel near the top of your mat so that it's there when you're ready.

- Prepare your strap or belt, which will be wrapped around your thighs when you've placed your block or ball between the knees. You want to make sure that the strap doesn't cut off circulation and that it's just tight enough on your thighs to keep your knees from falling open. Your legs should be able to stay upright and slightly closed without any effort at all.

- Lie down on the mat and shimmy the strap around your thighs, with the block or ball between your bent knees. Feet should be flat on the floor, hip-width apart and a comfortable distance from your buttocks, with your arms resting on the sides of your body.

- Adjust your body so that you feel comfortable in this pose, adding a rolled-up towel under your neck and/or head so that your muscles are soft and supple.

- Inhale and exhale as you progressively release your body weight into the ground, noticing which limbs are heavier and where the tension may be holding or gripping.

- Breath by breath, let go into the ground. Trust that your props will support you. Know that you are being held safely.

- Continue letting go of all the muscles of your thighs, back, neck, and face.

- Feel the weight of your head dropping into the floor and imagine that the arch of your lower back softens and moves toward the floor.

- Continue breathing and imagine that your breath softens and unravels any tightness that you may feel.

- For the last few minutes of this pose, let your hands come up to your belly, and imagine that the energy from them is soothing all of the hardworking cells that create your immunity, serotonin, and nervous-system relaxation chemicals.

- Slowly transition out of this pose by taking the ball or block from between your legs and sliding your strap off.

- Gently move around in any way that your body feels comfortable. Notice the changes in your muscle tone and energy.

- Mindfully roll to your side, carefully press yourself up into a sitting position, and notice the changes to your mind, body, and breath.

Supported
Child's Pose

*Good for: chronic pain, headaches, joint pain,
nerve pain, releasing tension, stress relief*

Feelings can float to the surface during times of stress. Taking a moment to pause, breathe, and reset helps your body process all the emotions that you may be feeling. This is an opportunity to find clarity and peace in the midst of chaos. This pose can be done seated at a chair and draped over a bed, or kneeling on the ground.

Props: Bolsters, bed pillows, and a large stack of blankets or towels that can be folded to adjust for deep comfort as you move into this pose.

Let's begin.

- Fold five blankets so that each is 8 to 12 inches wide, and long enough to support your torso and head when you fold forward. You may also use a bolster or bed pillows. Make sure that you have your pile close at hand as you begin.

- Sit astride the stack of blankets, or bolster with knees or feet resting on the floor (feet flat on the floor if you're sitting in a chair). Stay here a moment, readjusting your knees and feet so that you're completely comfortable.

- As you bend forward, place enough towels and pillows in front of you so that your stomach and chest will be gently supported when you bend over them.

- As you sit on the blankets or chair, imagine that your energy rises up to your heart, opening your collarbones so that the front of your body feels long and spacious.

- Deepen your breath and soften your jaw, eyes, and skin. Invite feelings of compassion and tenderness to move in through your tissue, bones, and blood vessels, and then into your core.

- Inhale as you stretch your spine toward the sky and then exhale as you fold from the hips, allowing your torso to settle on the blankets or pillows.

Restorative Legs-Elevated Pose

Good for: chronic pain, headaches, releasing tension, stress relief

In this pose, the legs rest while the whole body releases tension. This pose can relieve anxiety and mild depression, and regulate blood pressure while gently stretching the hamstrings, torso, and neck muscles. This is a wonderful way to increase diaphragmatic breathing and open up the chest muscles. This exercise is modified to use a couch or chair—the same exercise can be done 12 inches away from a wall with a bolster beneath the small of the back and the legs up the wall.

Contraindications: Serious neck or back conditions, menstruation, pregnancy after first trimester, glaucoma

Props: Chair, couch, or ottoman; two small towels for head and neck support; a bolster or rolled blankets to lift the hips up

Let's begin.

- To set up this pose, you'll need to find a space that allows you to lie on the floor with your legs supported on a couch, ottoman, or chair. If getting on the floor is difficult, you can use pillows to support your legs while you lie in bed.

- Gently lower yourself to the floor.

- Roll on to your back as you bring your legs up onto the chair with your knees bent. Rest your legs on the chair, couch, or ottoman, making sure they are supported and comfortable.

- If you need neck support, place a rolled towel or pillow under your neck and a small, folded towel under the head. Your head should be neutral with your chin, just slightly moving toward your chest.

- Rest your hands by your sides, on your belly, or on pillows.

- Make any adjustments you need to ensure you are comfortable.

- Take several long breaths as you progressively release all your body weight into the ground, letting your skin, muscles, and bones become heavy and relaxed.

- Rest here for 5 to 15 minutes.

- To come out of the pose, bring your knees toward your belly and roll to your side, making your arm into a pillow under your head.

- Take your time to come to a comfortable, seated position and close your practice by taking slow and easy breaths, noticing a difference in your body, mind, and breath.

Supported Bridge Pose

Good for: chronic pain, releasing tension

This supported back extension helps open the chest for better breathing and relieve the hunched posture that can come from sitting too long. The supportive nature of this exercise comes from the head and neck being lower than the heart, which promotes this parasympathetic system of "rest and digest."

Suggested breath: Feel into the lateral movement of your lungs and ribs during inhalation and exhalation, focusing breath on any area of the body that may feel stress, tension, or discomfort.

Props: Couch cushions, blankets, small pillows, eye pillow or an elastic bandage wrap to cover your eyes

Let's begin.

- Line up the couch pillows that will be supporting your legs and lower back, and a thinner pillow that will support your neck and head. If you don't have any neck or shoulder problems, feel free to allow the upper body and head to lie on the floor without a pillow.

- Place two rolled-up blankets, towels, or bed pillows to your side to support your arms if you have any nerve or shoulder pain. You can also allow the arms to be at your sides, palms up.

- Place yourself on the pillows and blankets, and cover your eyes via your preferred method.

- You may need a small pillow to support your head and neck, being mindful not to bend your head excessively forward to keep the vessels of the neck from becoming compressed. Your head should be below your shoulders in this position to achieve the greatest benefit.

- Feel the length in the back of the neck and the heaviness of your jaw, allowing your tongue to float freely in your mouth. Soften the backs of your eyes. If you notice any areas of gripping, tension, or tightness, allow them to soften with your breath as though the tension is a sugar cube dissolving in hot liquid.

- Use your breath, imagination, and awareness to release any area of tightness, discomfort, and disease, and give yourself permission to move deeply into a state of calm relaxation.

- Stay in this position for 3 to 15 minutes, imagining that your muscles are supple and relaxed, while at the same time easily and gently supporting your bones.

Crocodile Pose for Basic Diaphragmatic Breathing

Good for: chronic pain, releasing tension, stress relief

This is the best posture for sensing the flow of the breath. When you are lying facedown and are well supported, your body will naturally begin to breathe in a diaphragmatic way. This is a wonderful pose to use when you are nervous or feel tightness in your belly. Many people carry tension in their abdomens without their knowledge—this pose offers a chance to unblock the breath and release pent-up tension.

Props: One blanket or pillow; an eye pillow, band, or scarf that can be wrapped around your head

- Fold the blanket three times lengthwise to make a long, narrow blanket. It should be six to eight inches wide and no more than three inches thick. You can also use a pillow that is the length of your torso.

- Lie over the blanket or pillow so that it is under your abdomen and chest.

- Make a pillow of your arms or hands, or find a soft pillow and rest your head to either side. If this is uncomfortable for your neck, roll a small washcloth up and place it under your forehead so that you're able to breathe and your nose isn't squished.

- You may turn your feet in, with legs resting relatively close together, or turn them out, separating the legs until the inner thighs rest comfortably on the floor.

- If your head is turned to the side, place your eye pillow, band, or scarf over your eyes as best as you can. If your head is facedown, you can place an eye pillow over the back of your neck.

- Breathe deeply through your nose, making your exhale a little bit longer than your inhale. The idea is to quiet the pace of your thoughts by inhaling and exhaling and focusing on the rhythm of your breath.

- As you rest in this pose, become aware of how your breath moves through your body. The breath will find its own pace without you having to control the speed. Just let the body breathe.

- Now bring your awareness to your abdomen and feel how it presses against the floor or the pillow as you inhale, and recedes as you exhale. Relax the muscles in your belly, and let these movements of the abdomen become deep and soothing.

- Shift your attention to the sides of the rib cage. Notice how the lower ribs expand laterally with the inhalation and contract with the exhalation. The rib cage expands as the diaphragm contracts, and the ribs return inward as the diaphragm relaxes.

- Finally, bring your attention to your lower back. Notice that as you inhale, the back rises, and as you exhale, the back falls. Soften your back muscles and allow the breath to flow without resistance. This is a particularly relaxing sensation, and you may find that it helps relieve lower back tension that is often difficult to release.

- Remain resting in crocodile pose while you feel the breath around your midsection. Notice how relaxed your breathing has become.

- When you feel refreshed, come out of this posture slowly, creating a smooth transition back to normal breathing. Notice the changes in your body, mind, and breath.

Reclining
Bound-Angle Pose

Good for: chronic pain, releasing tension, stress relief

This pose is thought to be one of the most important of the restorative series. It allows for deep opening with safety and support. This pose is excellent to use before bed to release worrisome thoughts of the day, to ground and center, and to prepare your body for the restoration of sleep.

You will experience a gentle opening of the hips and chest with a focus on breathing, while reducing stress and tension and decreasing the anxiety that accompanies chronic pain. When lying in this pose, you may be reminded of being cradled in the womb. The setup for this pose is extensive, and many people use it as one long, 30-minute meditative pose.

Contraindications: Pregnancy after the first trimester; knee injury; diagnosed disc disease; intense pain in neck, lower back, or knees. Pillows can be used to support joints that are stiff and painful.

Props: Pillows, blankets, and bolsters to prop up the torso, hips, and knees; a yoga belt or heavy sandbag; ankle or wrist weights; eye pillow or scarf; timer

Let's begin.

- Stack pillows, blankets, or bolsters as a base of support for the upper chest. A 36-inch foam roller works well if you don't have access to a yoga bolster.

- Make sure you have your props close at hand—stacks of pillows that will support your knees as they flop open, and blankets to put under your head as well as on top of your body for deep relaxation.

- Sit in front of the short end of your bolster with it touching your tailbone. Bend your knees and place your feet on the floor, using your arms for support as you gently lie down. The bolster should support your sacrum through to your head. Adjust the height of the bolster or stack of blankets so that your back feels comfortable. You should have a stack of blankets that props up your upper back.

- Make sure that your neck is adequately supported with a small pillow or folded towels or a blanket. Your head should not be too high or low—your forehead should be higher than your chin, your chin higher than your breastbone, and your breastbone higher than your pubic bone. Once positioned, your torso should be at a 45-degree angle to the floor.

- Place the soles of your feet together and let your knees fall to the sides.

- Place a long, rolled blanket or pillow under each outer thigh, making sure that there is no effort in your hip sockets. The weight of your legs should be completely supported.

- The point of the pose is not to stretch the inner thighs, but to relax the abdomen and open the chest. As you relax, your feet may slide away from you. To use a belt to keep your feet in place, fasten it into a loop long enough to accommodate the distance from your hips to your feet while lying down. You may need to use two belts, together. Bring the belt over your head and position it around your hips. With the soles of your feet together, wrap the free side of the loop around your feet and be careful that the buckle does not press into your skin.

- Place two long, rolled blankets or pillows to support your forearms, and lie down again.

- Make sure that you have no tension in your shoulders and that your wrists and elbows feel supported.

- Place an eye pillow or scarf over your eyes.

CONTINUED

- As you settle in, allow the props to support your body so that it becomes effortless. Don't try to relax—allow the breath to move through you and the props to do the work.

- Begin with the centering breath, a slow, gentle inhalation followed by a slow, gentle exhalation. Follow this with several normal breaths in whatever way feels natural.

- Follow with more of the centering breath by slowly inviting the inhalation to move more deeply into your body. Let the air come to you. As you inhale, imagine that the breath is breathing you. Allow your intention to follow the inhalation and exhalation with gentle awareness. Begin to notice the quality and texture of your breath. With each cycle, allow your breath to become more and more refined and more nurturing, releasing any and all restrictions that it may encounter.

- At any time, resume normal breathing to come back to a quiet place of being if you find that centering breathing has moved you away from it.

- As you come back, let the outside world come into your awareness. Become aware of the sounds around you and the sensations of your body. Gently move around, stretching comfortably. When you're ready, remove your eye pillow or scarf and slowly blink your eyes open.

- Come up by pressing down with your arms and sitting up slowly. Undo the belts or remove the sandbag from your feet, and stretch your legs out in front of you to release any tension that might have occurred in your knees.

Supported Sequence

Good for: chronic pain, headaches, nerve pain, releasing tension, stress relief

This four-pose sequence allows you to surrender and reconnect to your deep, intuitive wisdom.

Suggested breath: Feel into the lateral movement of your lungs and ribs during inhalation and exhalation, focusing breath on any area of the body that may feel stress, tension, or discomfort.

Props: Yoga block or small stack of books, bolster, foam roller covered with a towel, couch cushions, and optional blanket. You can use two bed pillows to support the arms in these poses if you have any nerve or shoulder pain.

Supported Forward Fold

- Place a folded blanket underneath your buttocks to help tilt the pelvis forward and create length in the spine.

- Place a bolster or a thick pillow on top of your thighs.

- Place a block or six to eight inches of books on top of your bolster.

- Let the legs completely relax and let the feet splay out to the sides of your blanket in a position of ease.

- On an exhaled breath, let the chest melt down and allow the forehead to rest on the block.

- Notice the tops of your shoulders and invite them to soften and lengthen down as the back opens and relaxes.

- Breathe naturally in and out, being aware of how the breath fills your back and softens your tissues as you notice your relaxation.

CONTINUED

Supported Sequence *CONTINUED*

- Stay in this position for three to five minutes.

- Imagine that your body is softening into the pose as you are draped over the pillow, releasing any tension or thoughts with your breath.

Supported Wide-Leg Forward Fold

- Keep the bolster between your legs, connecting with the center of your body lengthwise. Open your legs to a comfortable V-shape. Keep the block or books on the top of the bolster, making sure it's high enough to keep your low back and neck comfortable.

- As you inhale, allow your spine to reach up toward the ceiling, finding length in the back of your body.

- As you exhale, let your chest melt over the bolster and let your forehead connect with the block or the books.

- Stay in this position for three to five minutes. Imagine that your muscles are melting as you lie draped over your bolster. If you notice any tight areas in your back, neck, or shoulders, imagine that those tight spots are like a sugar cube slowly dissolving with the heat of your breath.

Supported Supine Spinal Twist

- Remove the bolster from your belly and put it behind the body lengthwise in the middle of your blanket.

- From a seated position, bend both knees, and let them flop over to your right side of the body.

- Bring the bolster or pillow directly in line with your right hip.

- On an exhaled breath, let the chest melt over the bolster and bring your left ear to the bolster. Notice any tension that you may feel around your eyes. Imagine that the backs of your eyes are softening and that your gaze becomes gentle and soft.

- If it feels comfortable, for an added twist, switch the position of your head, bringing the right ear to the bolster and ensuring that there is no tension and no gripping.

- Stay in this position for three to five minutes and repeat on the other side.

Supported Savasana

- This pose tends to be the favorite part of any yoga practice. It's often called corpse pose, and allows your body completion and surrender.

- Lie down with your knees bent and feet flat, and move your bolster so that it is directly under your knees. You can relax your knees and extend your legs, or if you have low back pain, you may find that keeping them bent with the soles of the feet on the floor is more comfortable.

- Place a small blanket, folded towel, or small pillow underneath your head.

- Arms can rest at the side with the palms facing up, and you can use a bed pillow to support both arms if you have any nerve or shoulder pain.

CONTINUED

Supported Sequence *CONTINUED*

....

- Close your eyes, and feel them soften toward the back. Take a deep breath in and let go. Take another huge deep breath and exhale everything out.

- Notice the softening of your muscles as they melt into the floor, feeling your diaphragm rise easily and fall easily with your breath. Notice thoughts that may come and go without judgment.

- Stay in this position for 5 to 15 minutes.

*The good news
is that this complex
relationship between
the mind and the body
also allows you to
intervene in a positive
way to impact your
health and resilience.*

CHAPTER SEVEN

Continued Success

Congratulations on finishing this book. I know it's been quite a journey for you, but I hope it's one you'll continue in your quest for pain relief. In this chapter we will review all of the techniques you've learned and outline plans for your continued success.

The Path Forward

The mind and the body are powerful allies. The MBC shows us that our thoughts, feelings, beliefs, and attitudes affect how we function. If you have chronic pain, you might become depressed, anxious, and stressed. This constant worry or stress can cause tense muscles, pain, and stomach problems, as well as high blood pressure and other serious health conditions.

But the good news is that this complex relationship between the mind and the body also allows you to intervene in a positive way to impact your health and resilience. Negative thoughts and emotions can keep your brain from producing the chemicals that help heal your body. This doesn't mean that you're causing this issue. It just means that your body's default is the fight-or-flight mode, and it is wired to be aware of all the negative stressful things in life in order to stay safe. This is just your basic wiring, and you have to go in and tinker with it in order to change it.

In order to change it, you have to become aware of the fact that it isn't working correctly. Positive and happy memories don't naturally stick in the brain. You have to do something to wire them in so that you can benefit from having positive, healing chemicals in your brain. The MBC exercises in this book are designed to help you rewire your brain for happiness, well-being, and health.

Your thoughts and emotions create a chemical language that communicates with your brain, peripheral nervous system, organs, and immune and endocrine systems. Becoming aware of how all these systems work together is essential for you to make the necessary changes to address your pain and create balance in your life. You have a pharmacy of chemicals that can decrease your pain, help you sleep, and allow you to learn the unique language of your body. Like any new language, learning all the nuances and special rules about the MBC takes time and experimentation to get right. The concept of MBC has been around for hundreds of years, yet it's not what we automatically think about when we have pain and stress. A good friend of mine tells me that "inch by inch, life's a cinch." I take that to mean that change will happen in time if we give it a chance.

MBC Review Techniques

In the previous chapters, you've learned five mind-body connection tools to help you with managing and befriending your pain.

Reframing is a powerful coping technique that allows you the opportunity to change how you think about pain and stress. This MBC tool affects your body's chemistry and your ability to thrive, rather than to just survive. The exercises in this book help you become aware of your thoughts in order to change them and achieve the ultimate goal of being able to move into your life with renewed purpose.

Mindfulness is also a coping strategy for stress and pain. Research shows us that practicing mindfulness allows us to listen to our body and heart in a more intuitive way. It's about paying attention to the present moment without any judgment. This is a practice that takes time to cultivate and can be done on the fly in any circumstance once you've created the habit of this way of being present. Part of the mindful experience is not that we are paying attention, it's about *how* we pay attention.

Meditation is a deeper form of paying attention. It includes a mindfulness component, yet it's more structured and done for a set period of time. Included are guided meditations, walking meditations, and just being present with yourself. Purposeful coloring or painting can be a meditative practice.

Breathwork is most commonly used for insomnia and pain, and is the common thread through all the MBC exercises. There are a variety of breathing exercises that help you connect your body and mind in a harmonious way.

Restorative yoga combines gentle and supported movement with mindfulness, meditation, and breathwork. Each pose requires a focus on the breath, calming the mind and releasing thoughts, fears, and expectations.

Future Game Plan

Learning new skills requires finding ways to create habits. To change a habit means that you actually have to do the thing that changes your habit. Finding the right tool that you will use on a daily basis is the key to creating sustainable change. There are many useful apps for journaling, meditation, pain management, and more. But make sure that the app is transparent with its privacy settings. Apps make money selling your information, so make sure that you've kept it private.

My favorite method is to set timers on my phone that tell me exactly what I should be doing when the timer goes off. I've suggested that my patients set a timer to check in with their breath, mind, and body. You can create any affirmation that you want to look at, and set the timer for as many times a day as you want. Forty-seven percent of people spend most of their waking hours thinking about something other than what they're doing. If you're one of them, this can help you get back into your body, and start making habits that can change how you think and feel, and ultimately reduce your pain.

Final Words of Encouragement

Anyone who has chronic pain knows that it changes your life. It's a multidimensional condition that affects your body, emotions, mind, and spirit. MBC allows you the freedom to learn new behaviors and skills to navigate the complexities that your persistent pain presents to you on a day-to-day basis.

Avoiding pain is a hard habit to break. Many of the exercises in this book ask you to move into your body and into your pain. This takes trust. And in order to teach your body to trust movement and change, time and experimentation are needed to find the right fit. Be kind to yourself, because pain is real and only you know what it feels like to have that experience. Only you know what it will take to change an attitude, a feeling, or a belief.

Be creative with the exercises and understand that what feels good one day may not feel good the next. Your body's natural inclination is to heal. Using the MBC exercises in this book will allow your body to access its natural ability to heal. I invite you to trust the process and begin your journey of healing.

Resources

Articles

Harvard Health Publishing. "Yoga for Pain Relief." Harvard Medical School. April 2015. health.Harvard.edu/alternative-and-complementary -medicine/yoga-for-pain-relief.

Hayes, Kim. "Medication Errors More Than Double. "AARP. July 24, 2017. AARP.org/health/drugs-supplements/info-2017/medication -errors-rise-fd.html.

Jones, Michael. "Pain and How You Sense It." myDr. Last modified February 29, 2012. myDr.com.au/pain/pain-and-how-you-sense-it.

Kos, Blaze. "Cognitive reframing – it's not about what happens to you, but how you frame it." agileleanlife.com/cognitive-reframing.

McGonigal, Kelly. "Restorative Yoga for Chronic Pain." Yoga International. 2009. YogaInternational.com/article/view/restorative -yoga-for-chronic-pain.

Sipherd, Ray. "The Third-Leading Cause of Death in US Most Doctors Don't Want You to Know About." CNBC. February 22, 2018. CNBC .com/2018/02/22/medical-errors-third-leading-cause-of-death-in -america.html.

Books

Amen, Daniel G. *Change Your Brain, Change Your Life: The Breakthrough Program for Conquering Anxiety, Depression, Obsessiveness, Lack of Focus, Anger, and Memory Problems*. New York: Harmony Books, 2015.

Braden, Gregg. *Resilience From the Heart: The Power to Thrive in Life's Extremes*. Carlsbad, CA: Hay House, 2014.

Braden, Gregg. *The Spontaneous Healing of Belief: Shattering the Paradigm of False Limits*. Carlsbad, CA: Hay House, 2008.

Brown, Brené. *Daring Greatly: How the Courage to Be Vulnerable Transforms the Way We Live, Love, Parent, and Lead.* New York: Avery, 2012.

Butler, David, and Lorimer Moseley. *The Explain Pain Handbook Protectometer.* Adelaide, South Australia: NOI Group, 2015.

Butler, David, and Lorimer Moseley. *Explain Pain Supercharged: The Clinician's Handbook.* Adelaide, South Australia: NOI Group, 2017.

Carlson, Richard, and Joseph Bailey. *Slowing Down to the Speed of Life: How to Create a More Peaceful, Simpler Life from the Inside Out.* New York: Harper Collins, 1997.

Childre, Doc, and Deborah Rozman. *Transforming Depression: The HeartMath Solution to Feeling Overwhelmed, Sad, and Stressed* Oakland CA: New Harbinger Publications, 2007.

Chopra, Deepak. *The Way of the Wizard: Twenty Spiritual Lessons for Creating the Life You Want.* New York: Harmony Books, 1995.

Dispenza, Joe. *Breaking the Habit of Being Yourself: How to Lose Your Mind and Create a New One.* Carlsbad, CA: Hay House, 2012.

Dispenza, Joe. *You Are the Placebo: Making Your Mind Matter.* Carlsbad, CA: Hay House, 2014.

Dossey, Larry. *One Mind: How Our Individual Mind Is Part of a Greater Consciousness and Why It Matters.* Carlsbad, CA: Hay House, 2013.

Emmons, Henry. *The Chemistry of Calm: A Powerful, Drug-Free Plan to Quiet Your Fears and Overcome Your Anxiety.* New York: Atria Paperback, 2010.

Emmons, Henry. *The Chemistry of Joy: A Three Step Program for Overcoming Depression through Western Science and Eastern Wisdom.* New York: Fireside, 2006.

Fairfield, Peter. *Deep Happy: How to Get There and Always Find Your Way Back.* San Francisco, CA: Red Wheel/Weiser, 2012.

Finley, Guy. *The Essential Laws of Living Fearless: Find the Power to Never Feel Powerless Again.* San Francisco, CA: Red Wheel/Weiser, 2008.

Gilbert, Elizabeth. *Big Magic: Creative Living beyond Fear.* New York: Riverhead Books, 2015.

Grout, Pam. *E-Squared: Nine Do-It-Yourself Energy Experiments That Prove Your Thoughts Create Your Reality.* Carlsbad, CA: Hay House, 2014.

Hansen, Rick. *Buddha's Brain: The Practical Neuroscience of Happiness, Love, and Wisdom.* Oakland, CA: New Harbinger Publications, 2009.

Hansen, Rick. *Hardwiring Happiness: The New Brain Science of Contentment, Calm, and Confidence.* New York: Harmony, 2013.

Martin, Paul. *The Healing Mind: The Vital Links between Brain and Behavior, Immunity and Disease.* New York: Thomas Dunne Books, 1997.

Maté, Garbor. *When the Body Says No: Understanding the Stress-Disease Connection.* Hoboken, NJ: John Wiley and Sons. 2003.

McEwen, Bruce, and Elizabeth Norton Lasley. *The End of Stress as We Know It.* New York: Dana Press, 2002.

Pearsall, Paul. *The Heart's Code: Tapping the Wisdom and Power of Our Heart Energy.* New York: Broadway Books, 1998.

Pert, Candace, B. *Molecules of Emotion: The Science behind Mind-Body Medicine.* New York: Touchstone, 1999.

Ruiz, Don Miguel. *The Mastery of Love: A Practical Guide to the Art of Relationship.* San Rafael, CA: Amber-Allen Publishing, 1999.

Sapolsky, Robert M. *Why Zebras Don't Get Ulcers: The Acclaimed Guide to Stress, Stress-Related Diseases, and Coping.* New York: Times Books, 2004.

Seaward, Brian Luke. *Managing Stress: Principles and Strategies for Health and Well-Being.* 8th ed. Burlington, MA: Jones and Bartlett Learning, 2015.

Seaward, Brian Luke. *Quiet Mind, Fearless Heart: The Taoist Path through Stress and Spirituality.* Hoboken, NJ: John Wiley and Sons, 2005.

Seaward, Brian Luke. *Stand Like Mountain, Flow Like Water: Reflections on Stress and Human Spirituality.* Deerfield Beach, FL: Health Communications, 2007.

Small, Gary, and Gigi Vorgan. *2 Weeks to a Younger Brain: An Innovative Program for a Better Memory and a Sharper Mind.* West Palm Beach, FL: Humanix Books, 2016.

Tolle, Eckhart. *A New Earth: Awakening to Your Life's Purpose.* New York: Plume, 2006.

Tolle, Eckhart. *The Power of Now: A Guide to Spiritual Enlightenment.* Vancouver, Canada: Namaste Publishing, 2004.

References

Benor, Daniel. "TWR Method." *Daniel Benor, MD.* Accessed August 3, 2020. DanielBenor.com/twr-method.

Borsook, David. "A Future without Chronic Pain: Neuroscience and Clinical Research." *Cerebrum* 7 (2012). PubMed.ncbi.nlm.nih .gov/23447793.

Borysenko, Joan Z. "Too Much Holiday Stress?" *Heal Your Life.* November 13, 2015. HealYourLife.com/too-much-holiday-stress.

Bradt, Steve. "Wandering Mind Not a Happy Mind." *The Harvard Gazette.* November 11, 2010. news.Harvard.edu/gazette/story/2010/11 /wandering-mind-not-a-happy-mind.

Brower, Vicki. "Mind–Body Research Moves towards the Main-stream." *EMBO Reports* 7 (2006): 358–61. doi.org/10.1038/sj.embor .7400671.

Burke, Nikita N., David P. Finn, Brian E. McGuire, and Michelle Roche. "Psychological Stress in Early Life as a Predisposing Factor for the Development of Chronic Pain: Clinical and Pre-clinical Evidence and Neurobiological Mechanisms." *Journal of Neuroscience Research* 95, no., 6 (2017): 1257–70. doi.org/10.1002 /jnr.23802.

Busch, Volker, Walter Magerl, Uwe Kern, Joachim Haas, Göran Hajak, and Peter Eichhammer. "The Effect of Deep and Slow Breathing on Pain Perception, Autonomic Activity, and Mood Processing—An Experimental Study." *Pain Medicine* 13, no. 2 (February 2012): 215–28. doi.org/10.1111/j.1526-4637.2011.01243.x.

Cooke, Rachel. "'Sleep Should Be Prescribed': What Those Late Nights Out Could Be Costing You." September 24, 2017. TheGuardian .com/lifeandstyle/2017/sep/24/why-lack-of-sleep-health-worst-enemy -matthew-walker-why-we-sleep.

Coppens, E., P. Van Wambeke, B. Morlion, N. Weltens, H. Giao Ly, J. Tack, P. Luyten, and L. Van Oudenhove. "Prevalence and Impact of Childhood Adversities and Post-Traumatic Stress Disorder in Women with Fibromyalgia and Chronic Widespread Pain." *European Journal of Pain* 21, no. 9 (2017): 1582–90. doi.org/10.1002/ejp.1059.

Creswell, J. David, Adrienne A. Taren, Emily K. Lindsay, Carol M. Greco, Peter J. Gianaros, April Fairgrieve, Anna L. Marsland, Kirk Warren Brown, Baldwin M. Way, Rhonda K. Rosen, and Jennifer L. Ferris. "Alterations in Resting-State Functional Connectivity Link Mindfulness Meditation with Reduced Interleukin-6: A Randomized Controlled Trial." *Biological Psychiatry* 80, no. 1 (July 2016). doi .org/10.1016/j.biopsych.2016.01.008.

Dahlhamer, James, Jacqueline Lucas, Carla Zelaya, Richard Nahin, Sean Mackey, Lynn DeBar, Robert Kerns, Michael Von Korff, Linda Porter, and Charles Helmick. "Prevalence of Chronic Pain and High-Impact Chronic Pain Among Adults—United States, 2016." *Morbidity and Mortality Weekly Report* 67 (2018): 1001–1006. CDC .gov/mmwr/volumes/67/wr/mm6736a2.htm.

De Ruddere, Lies, Liesbet Goubert, Michaël André Louis Stevens, Myriam Deveugele, Kenneth Denton Craig, and Geert Crombez. "Health Care Professionals' Reactions to Patient Pain: Impact of Knowledge about Medical Evidence and Psychosocial Influences." *Journal of Pain* 15, no. 3 (2014): 262–70. doi.org/10.1016/j.jpain.2013.11.002.

Denk, Franziska, Stephen B. McMahon, and Irene Tracey. "Pain Vulnerability: A Neurobiological Perspective." *Nature Neuroscience* 17 (2014): 192–200. doi.org/10.1038/nn.3628.

Dhanvijay, Anupkumar, Angesh Harish Bagade, Arbind Kumar Choudhary, Sadawarte Sahebrao Kishanrao, and Nitin Dhokne. "Alternate Nostril Breathing and Autonomic Function in Healthy Young Adults." *IOSR Journal of Dental and Medical Sciences* 14, no. 3 (2015). ResearchGate.net/publication/274070158_Alternate_Nostril_Breathing _and_Autonomic_Function_in_Healthy_Young_Adults.

Doll, Anselm, Britta K. Hölzel, Satja Mulej Bratec, Christine C. Boucard, Xiyao Xie, Afra M. Wohlschläger, and Christian Sorg. "Mindful Attention to Breath Regulates Emotions via Increased Amygdala-Prefrontal Cortex Connectivity." *NeuroImage* 134 (2016): 305–13. doi.org/10.1016/j.neuroimage.2016.03.041.

Fenton, Bradford W., Elim Shih, and Jessica Zolton. "The Neurobiology of Pain Perception in Normal and Persistent Pain." *Pain Management* 5, no. 4 (2015): 297–317. doi.org/10.2217/pmt.15.27.

Ferrari, Robert, and Deon Louw. "Correlation between Expectations of Recovery and Injury Severity Perception in Whiplash-Associated Disorders." *Journal of Zhejiang University Science B* 12, 8 (2011): 683–86. doi.org/10.1631/jzus.B1100097.

Ghiya, Shreya. "Alternate Nostril Breathing: A Systematic Review of Clinical Trials." *International Journal of Research in Medical Sciences* 5, no. 8 (2017). dx.doi.org/10.18203/2320-6012.ijrms20173523.

Goyal, Madhav, Sonal Singh, Erica M. S. Sibinga, et al. "Meditation Programs for Psychological Stress and Well-Being." *JAMA Internal Medicine* 174, no. 3 (2014): 357–68. doi.org/10.1001/jamainternmed .2013.13018.

Grace, Fran. "Viktor Frankl and the Search for Meaning: A Conversation with Alexander Vesely and Mary Cimiluca." *Daily Good.* April 14, 2017. DailyGood.org/story/1578/viktor-frankl-and-the-search-for -meaning-a-conversation-with-alexander-vesely-and-mary-cimiluca.

Green, Elmer, and Alyce Green. *Beyond Biofeedback.* Ft. Wayne, IN: Delacorte Press, 1977.

Grout, Pam. *E-Squared: Nine Do-It-Yourself Energy Experiments That Prove Your Thoughts Create Your Reality.* Carlsbad, CA: Hay House, 2014.

Hall, Jo, Stephen Kellett, Raul Berrios, Manreesh Kaur Bains, and Shonagh Scott. "Efficacy of Cognitive Behavioral Therapy for Generalized Anxiety Disorder in Older Adults: Systematic Review,

Meta-Analysis, and Meta-Regression." *American Journal of Geriatric Psychiatry* 24, no 11 (2016): 1063–73. doi.org/10.1016/j.jagp.2016.06.006.

Hạnh Thích Nhất. "Living without Stress or Fear: Essential Teachings on the True Source of Happiness." Louisville, CO: Sounds True, 2009.

Hedblom, Marcus, Bengt Gunnarsson, Behzad Iravani, Igor Knez, Martin Schaefer, Pontus Thorsson, and Johan N. Lundström. "Reduction of Physiological Stress by Urban Green Space in a Multi-Sensory Virtual Experiment." *Scientific Reports* 9 (2019). Nature.com/articles/s41598-019-46099-7.

Holman, Andrew J. "Positional Cervical Spinal Cord Compression and Fibromyalgia: A Novel Comorbidity with Important Diagnostic and Treatment Implications." *Journal of Pain* 9, no. 7 (2008): 613–22. doi.org/10.1016/j.jpain.2008.01.339.

Jerath, Ravinder, Molly W. Crawford, Vernon A. Barnes, and Kyler Harden. "Self-Regulation of Breathing as a Primary Treatment for Anxiety." *Applied Psychophysiology and Biofeedback* 40, no. 2 (2015): 107–15. doi.org/10.1007/s10484-015-9279-8.

Kabat-Zinn, Jon. *Full Catastrophe Living: Using the Wisdom of Your Body and Mind to Face Stress, Pain, and Illness.* New York: Bantam Books, 2013.

Khoury, Samar, Marjo H. Piltonen, Anh-Tien Ton, Tiffany Cole, Alexander Samoshkin, Shad B. Smith, Inna Belfer, Gary D. Slade, Roger B. Fillingim, Joel D. Greenspan, Richard Ohrbach, William Maixner, G. Gregory Neely, Adrian W. R. Serohijos, and Luda Diatchenko. "A Functional Substitution in the L-Aromatic Amino Acid Decarboxylase Enzyme Worsens Somatic Symptoms via a Serotonergic Pathway." *Annals of Neurology* 86, no. 2 (June 2019). doi.org/10.1002/ana.25521.

Kircanski, Katharina, Monica Wu, and John Piacentini. "Reduction of Subjective Distress in CBT for Childhood OCD: Nature of Change,

Predictors, and Relation to Treatment Outcome." *Journal of Anxiety Disorders* 28, no. 2 (2014): 125–32. doi.org/10.1016/j.janxdis.2013.05.004.

Kirkley, Alexandra, Trevor B. Birmingham, Robert B. Litchfield, J. Robert Giffin, Kevin R. Willits, Cindy J. Wong, Brian G. Feagan, Allan Donner, Sharon H. Griffin, Linda M. D'Ascanio, Janet E. Pope, and Peter J. Fowler. "A Randomized Trial of Arthroscopic Surgery for Osteoarthritis of the Knee." *New England Journal of Medicine* 359, no. 11 (2008): 1097–1107. doi.org/10.1056/NEJMoa0708333.

Kurt, Münevver, Melahat Akdeniz, and Ethem Kavukcu. "Assessment of Comorbidity and Use of Prescription and Nonprescription Drugs in Patients Above 65 Years Attending Family Medicine Outpatient Clinics." *Gerontology and Geriatric Medicine* 5 (2019). doi.org/10.1177/2333721419874274.

Lasselin, Julie, Mike K. Kemani, Marie Kanstrup, Gunnar L. Olsson, John Axelsson, Anna Andreasson, Mats Lekander, and Rikard K. Wicksell. "Low-Grade Inflammation May Moderate the Effect of Behavioral Treatment for Chronic Pain in Adults." *Journal of Behavioral Medicine* 39, no. 5 (2016): 916–24. doi.org/10.1007/s10865-016-9769-z.

Laupattarakasem, Wiroon, Malinee Laopaiboon, Pisamai. Laupattarakasem, and Chut Sumananont. "Arthroscopic Debridement for Knee Osteoarthritis." *Cochrane Database of Systematic Reviews* (2008). doi.org/10.1002/14651858.CD005118.pub2.

Levine, Steven. *Healing into Life and Death.* New York: Anchor, 1987.

Louw, Adriaan, Ina Diener, Merrill R. Landers, Kory Zimney, and Emilio J. Puentedura. "Three-Year Follow-Up of a Randomized Controlled Trial Comparing Preoperative Neuroscience Education for Patients Undergoing Surgery for Lumbar Radiculopathy." *Journal of Spine Surgery* 2, no. 4 (2016): 289–98. doi.org/10.21037/jss.2016.12.04

Louw, Adriaan, Jessie Podalak, Kory Zimney, Stephen Schmidt, and Emilio J. Puentedura. "Can Pain Beliefs Change in Middle School

Students? A Study of the Effectiveness of Pain Neuroscience Education." *Physiotherapy: Theory and Practice* 34, no. 7 (2018): 542–50. doi.org/10.1080/09593985.2017.1423142.

Louw, Adriaan, Kory Zimney, Christine O'Hotto, and Sandra Hilton. "The Clinical Application of Teaching People about Pain." *Physiotherapy: Theory and Practice* 32, no. 5 (2016): 385–95. doi.org/10.1080 /09593985.2016.1194652.

Lucas, Alexander R., Heidi D. Klepin, Stephen W. Porges, and W. Jack Rejeski. "Mindfulness-Based Movement: A Polyvagal Perspective." *Integrative Cancer Therapies* 17, no. 1 (2018): 5–15. doi .org/10.1177/1534735416682087.

Lundin, John. "Meditation—Taming Your Monkey Mind." *Medium.* February 27, 2018. Medium.com/@johnlundin/meditation-taming-your-monkey-mind-f0ba9bd50e95.

Mariotti, Agnese. "The Effects of Chronic Stress on Health: New Insights into the Molecular Mechanisms of Brain-Body Communication." *Future Science OA* 1, no. 3 (2015). doi.org/10.4155/fso.15.21.

McBeth J., A. J. Silman, A. Gupta, Y. H. Chiu, D. Ray, R. Morriss, C. Dickens, Y. King, and G. J. Macfarlane. "Moderation of Psychosocial Risk Factors through Dysfunction of the Hypothalamic-Pituitary -Adrenal Stress Axis in the Onset of Chronic Widespread Musculoskeletal Pain: Findings of a Population-Based Prospective Cohort Study." *Arthritis & Rheumatism* 56, no. 1 (2007): 360–71. doi.org /10.1002/art.22336.

Mills, Sarah E. E., Karen P. Nicholson, and Blair Smith. "Chronic Pain: A Review of Its Epidemiology and Associated Factors in Population-Based Studies." *British Journal of Anaesthesia* 123, no. 2 (2019): e273–e283. doi.org/10.1016/j.bja.2019.03.023.

Mitchell, Marilyn. "Dr. Herbert Benson's Relaxation Response." *Psychology Today.* March 29, 2013. PsychologyToday.com/us/blog /heart-and-soul-healing/201303/dr-herbert-benson-s-relaxation -response.

Moseley, J. Bruce, Kimberly O'Malley, Nancy J. Petersen, Terri J. Menke, Baruch A. Brody, David H. Kuykendall, John C. Hollingsworth, Carol M. Ashton, and Nelda P. Wray. "A Controlled Trial of Arthroscopic Surgery for Osteoarthritis of the Knee." *New England Journal of Medicine* 347, no. 11 (2002): 81–88. doi.org/10.1056/NEJMoa013259.

National Institute of Mental Health. "Any Anxiety Disorder." National Institutes of Health. Last modified November 2017. NIMH.NIH.gov/health/statistics/any-anxiety-disorder.shtml.

Papanicolas, Irene, Liana R. Woskie, and Ashish K. Jha. "Health Care Spending in the United States and Other High-Income Countries." *JAMA* 319, no. 10 (2018): 1024–39. doi.org/10.1001/jama.2018.1150.

Peper, Erik, and Fred Shaffer. "Biofeedback History: An Alternative View." *Biofeedback* 38 (2010): 142–47. doi.org/10.5298/1081-5937-38.4.03.

Pitcher, Mark H., Michael Von Korff, M. Catherine Bushnell, and Linda Porter. "Prevalence and Profile of High-Impact Chronic Pain in the United States." *The Journal of Pain* 20, no. 2 (2019): 146–60. doi.org/10.1016/j.jpain.2018.07.006.

Shahidi, Bahar, Douglas Curran-Everett, and Katrina S. Maluf. "Psychosocial, Physical, and Neurophysiological Risk Factors for Chronic Neck Pain: A Prospective Inception Cohort Study." *Journal of Pain* 16, no. 12 (2015): 1288–99. doi.org/10.1016/j.jpain.2015.09.002.

Smith, Toby O., Jack R. Dainty, Esther Williamson, and Kathryn R. Martin. "Association between Musculoskeletal Pain with Social Isolation and Loneliness: Analysis of the English Longitudinal Study of Ageing." *British Journal of Pain* 13, no. 2 (2019): 82–90. doi.org/10.1177/2049463718802868.

Sood, Amit, and David T. Jones. "On Mind Wandering, Attention, Brain Networks, and Meditation." *Explore* 9, no. 3 (2013): 136–41. doi.org/10.1016/j.explore.2013.02.005.

Srinivasan, T. M. "Bridging the Mind-Body Divide." *International Journal of Yoga* 6, no. 2 (2013): 85–86. doi.org/10.4103/0973 -6131.113389.

Synnott, Aoife, Mary O'Keeffe, Samantha Bunzli, Wim Dankaerts, Peter O'Sullivan, and Kieran O'Sullivan. "Physiotherapists May Stigmatise or Feel Unprepared to Treat People with Low Back Pain and Psychosocial Factors That Influence Recovery: A Systematic Review." *Journal of Physiotherapy* 61, no. 2 (2015): 68–76. doi.org/10.1016 /j.jphys.2015.02.016.

Tsai, H. J., Terry B. J. Kuo, Guo-She Lee, and Cheryl C. H. Yang. "Efficacy of Paced Breathing for Insomnia: Enhances Vagal Activity and Improves Sleep Quality." *Psychophysiology* 52, no. 3 (2015): 388–96. doi.org/10.1111/psyp.12333.

Twomey, Conal, Gary O'Reilly, and Michael Byrne. "Effectiveness of Cognitive Behavioural Therapy for Anxiety and Depression in Primary Care: A Meta-Analysis." *Family Practice* 32, no. 1 (2015): 3–15. doi.org/10.1093/fampra/cmu060.

Vigotsky, Andrew D., and Ryan P. Bruhns. "The Role of Descending Modulation in Manual Therapy and Its Analgesic Implications: A Narrative Review." *Pain Research and Treatment* (2015). doi.org /10.1155/2015/292805.

Wolpe, Joseph. *The Practice of Behavior Therapy.* New York: Pergamon Press, 1969.

Zeidan, Fadel, Katherine T. Martucci, Robert A. Kraft, Nakia S. Gordon, John G. McHaffie, and Robert C. Coghill. "Brain Mechanisms Supporting the Modulation of Pain by Mindfulness Meditation." *Journal of Neuroscience* 31, no. 14 (2011): 5540–48. doi.org/10.1523/JNEUROSCI.5791-10.2011.

Index

Acknowledgments

I want to give thanks to my patients who've inspired me to expand my education and to integrate mind-body medicine into my practice. They trust me with tender hearts, raw courage, and endless patience as we craft new blueprints for healing. I am humbled by the grace, dignity, and joy that I witness in people with persistent pain. Kahlil Gibran said, "Your joy can fill you only as deeply as your sorrow has carved you." My patients have taught me far more than I've ever taught them, and have made me a better clinician.

I am deeply grateful for the pain that drove me to find a path to self-care and resilience, and to my father, who showed me that you are never too old to learn new skills. I want to acknowledge and give thanks to my life partner, Steve, who has supported me in my lifetime commitment to education, training, and endless quantities of books.

About the Author

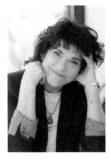

Anna McConville, DPT, PT, PNE, is a respected expert in the field of holistic physical therapy and chronic pain. She began her career as a professional mime and physical performer, which brings a unique perspective to her work as a therapist, author, and pain consultant. McConville began practicing meditation 40 years ago to heal from chronic pain, and this started her exploration into the field of mind-body medicine and self-healing. She integrates mindfulness, humor, and laughter in her telehealth pain programs. She helps her clients find creative solutions to reduce pain and understand their unique language of healing while teaching them how to access tools to live with less pain and greater resilience.

McConville has certifications in pain neuroscience, biofeedback, Pilates, Reiki, stress management, and more. She is a student of quantum physics and energy medicine, and is excited about the research that supports the premise that we can create a resilient life by changing our neural pathways. She loves to hike, bike, and camp, and fuels her creativity with nature, fiber art, and writing.

CPSIA information can be obtained
at www.ICGtesting.com
Printed in the USA
JSHW041557141120
9579JS00004B/4

9 781647 399511